This book is dedicated to my children. You inspire me every day in ways that I hope you can feel and understand one day.

Table of Contents

Forward

The challenge of ADD/ADHD (Attention Deficit Disorder or Attention Deficit Hyperactivity Disorder) is faced by millions of North Americans, and the total numbers will increase this year by millions. In facing my challenges head-on, I realized there were more books, web sites, papers, doctors, counselors, coaches, seminars and people out there than any human could possibly absorb, let alone decipher, especially adults with ADD.

This book has been written to share my experience of Adult ADD with whoever wants to experience it with me. It is also written for people with ADD, in that I realize the worst thing you can do to a person with ADD is tell them to read a 500 page book that drones on and on. This book is designed to try and hold your attention, to be simple to read and understand and most importantly, to share my experience and many of the resources I have found to be helpful. In reading this book you may simply be an interested party, you or your child, mother, friend or student may suffer from ADD. This book is about my personal experience. Please note that I am not a doctor nor am I offering medical or therapeutic advice. I wanted to tell as many people as I could, that the challenges of ADD can be met and overcome. What worked for me, may or may not work for you. It is important to adapt the ideas and tactics to fit your personality, learning and working styles. It will take a lot of effort and sacrifice, but that sacrifice and effort will pay off if you commit to it.

If sharing my experience can positively impact the direction of just one person who has ADD or knows someone who has ADD, then I will have accomplished what I set out to do.

Chapter 1. Attitude

"The longer I live, the more I realize the impact of attitude on life. Attitude to me, is more important than facts. It is more important than the past, than education, than money, than circumstances, than failures, than successes, than what other people think or say or do. It is more important than appearance, giftedness, or skill. It will make or break a company ... a church ... a home. The remarkable thing is we have a choice every day regarding the attitude we will embrace for that day. We cannot change the inevitable. The only thing we can do is play on the one string we have, and that is our attitude ... I am convinced that life is 10% what happens to me, and 90% how I react to it. And so it is with you, we are in charge of our Attitudes."
By Charles Swindoll.

As I pounded back what must have been my sixth or seventh scotch on top of a dozen beers already swirling in my stomach, I staggered by the bar and unknowingly bumped into a woman. With an over confident, smug attitude and a false sense of opinion on my favorite topic, me, I decided to offer the woman the privilege of a night with God's gift to women. My generous offer was not well received by her boyfriend who stood 6'6" and looked down on me at a humble 6'1" and 21 years of age. The standard exchange of young male testosterone enhanced with some rather foul adjectives filled the bar area and quickly I found myself outside, courtesy of the bouncers. With my attitude in tow and the stupidity of intoxication, I made my way back into the bar through an exit door. Soon enough, I found myself in more digressive exchanges with the woman's boyfriend.

Across the bar I spotted the woman and decided to approach her again. Through some miracle or perhaps the good that existed deep inside me, I apologized. The woman was gracious and very pleasant to me, as I recall. I was turning to walk away after saying good-bye, when the smash of the beer bottle could be heard as it shattered over my head. The boyfriend had decided to show me his displeasure about the earlier events and at the fact that I was talking to his girlfriend, again. As I pulled myself up off the floor, I disregarded my well being and became so enraged that adrenaline lifted me up and into battle resulting in a concussion. I remember grabbing a chair with which I hit him, throwing a beer bottle at him and tossing punches, some of which actually hit him. After the mayhem cleared, a cluster of patrons, bouncers, friends and strangers all filtered outside as the evening's events broke up. I headed to the hospital with a friend.

Did this guy completely over react? Absolutely. Were we both drunk and acting immaturely and foolishly? Yes. What was his problem? Why would he attack me like that? To this day, I don't really know the answer to those questions that pertain to him. However, I have the answers to the most important question; what about my conduct and attitude?

ADD impacted me in my youth, during college and as I became an adult. It wasn't until I was 36 years old that the true impact of ADD would result in my life crumbling, or so I thought. In an odd way, my life unraveling was a gift. A gift to me that had the potential to alter my life so dramatically and positively, that there was only one obstacle that stood in my way: my attitude.

The age old saying "attitude is everything" suddenly had new meaning to me. I never really understood it, felt it, or experienced it. In retrospect, I see that I had a horrible attitude and it was my attitude that would ultimately drive my life into a head on collision with the cold hard reality of my future.

All too often the best lessons in life are learned the hard way, especially for people affected by Attention Deficit Disorder (ADD). My mind has so much power and capability, its only limitation is my attitude. However, in reading about my experience please keep in mind that its purpose is to share and help others. In no way or form is this medical advice. Please consult your doctor to seek proper medical attention if you require it or know someone who does.

After experiencing so much in the last number of years in my life, it is also good to know that I'm not alone. There is an incredible list of notable people who have ***apparently*** battled ADD/ADHD, and I would say they have done very well in life if it is true. Such names that are linked to possibly having ADD/ADHD include:

-Ansel Adams (1902-1984) Photographer
-Ann Bancroft (1931-present) Actress
-Alexander Graham Bell (1862-1939) Telephone
  Inventor
-Harry Andersen (1952-present) Actor
-Hans Christian Anderson (1805-1875) Author
-Beethoven (1770-1827) Composer
-Harry Belafonte (1927-present) Actor, Vocalist
-Col. Gregory "Pappy" Boyington (1912-1988)
  WWII Flying Ace (Black Sheep Squadron Leader)
-Terry Bradshaw (1948-Present) Football QB
-Howie Mandel (1955-Present) Comedian
-George Burns (1896-1996) Actor
-Sir Richard Francis Burton (1821-1890)
-Explorer, Linguist, Scholar, Writer
-Admiral Richard Byrd (1888-1957) Aviator
-Thomas Carlyle (1795-1881) Scottish historian,
  critic, and sociological writer
-Andrew Carnegie (1835-1919) Industrialist
-Jim Carrey (1962-present) Comedian
-Lewis Carroll (1832-1898) Author (Alice in
  Wonderland)
-Prince Charles (1948-present) Future King
-Cher (1946-present) Actress/Singer
-Agatha Christie (1890-1976) Author
-Winston Churchill (1874-1965) Statesman (Failed
  the sixth grade)
-Bill Cosby (1937-present) Actor/Comedian
-Harvey Cushing M.D. (1869-1939) Greatest
  Neurosurgeon of the 20th Century
-Salvador Dali (1904-1989) Artist
-Leonardo da Vinci (1452-1519) Inventor, Artist
-John Denver (1943-1997) Musician
-Walt Disney (1901-1971)A newspaper editor fired
  him because he had "No good ideas"

-Kirk Douglas (1916-2004) Actor
-Thomas Edison (1847-1931) Inventor (His
  teachers told him he was too stupid to learn
  anything)
-Albert Einstein (1879-1955) Physicist
  (Einstein was four years old before he could
  Speak and seven before he could read)
-Dwight D. Eisenhower (1890-1969) U. S.
   President, Military General
-Michael Faraday (1791-1867) British Physicist &
  Chemist
-F. Scott Fitzgerald (1896-1940) Author
-Malcolm Forbes (1919-1990) Forbes Magazine
  Founder & Publisher
-Henry Ford (1863-1947) Automobile Innovator
-Benjamin Franklin (1706 - 1790) Politician
-Galileo (1564-1642) Mathematician/Astronomer
-Danny Glover (1947-present) Actor
-Tracey Gold (1969-present) Actress
-Whoopi Goldberg (1955-present) Actress
-George Frideric-Handel (1685-1759) Composer
-Valerie Hardin (1974-Present) Gothic Poet, Artist,
  Children's Author
-William Randolph Hearst (1863-1951)Newspaper
  Magnate
-Ernest Hemingway (1899-1961) Author
-Mariel Hemingway (1961-Present) Actress
-Milton Hershey "Chocolate King" (1857-1945)
-Dustin Hoffman (1937-Present) Actor
-Bruce Jenner (1949-Present) Athlete
-"Magic" Johnson (1959-present) Basketball Player
-Samuel Johnson (1709-1784) Author
-Michael Jordan (1963-present) Basketball Player
-John F. Kennedy (1917-1963) U. S. President
-Robert F. Kennedy (1925-1968) U.S. Senator
-Jason Kidd (1973-present) Basketball Player

-John Lennon (1940-1980) Musician
-Carl Lewis (1961-present) Olympic Gold Metalist
-Meriwether Lewis (Lewis & Clark) (1774 -1809)
  Explorer
-Abraham Lincoln (1809-1865) U.S. President
-Greg Louganis (1960-present) Olympic Gold
  Medalist (Diving)
-James Clerk Maxwell(1831-1879)British Physicist
-Steve McQueen (1930-1980) Actor
-Wolfgang Amadeus Mozart(1756-1791) Composer
-Napoleon Bonaparte (1769-1873) Emperor
-Nasser (Gamal Abdel-nasser) (1918-1970)
  Egyptian Leader
-Sir Issac Newton (1642-1727) Scientist &
  Mathematician (Did poorly in grade school)
-Nostradamus (1503-1566) Physician, Prophet
-Ozzy Osbourne (1948-present)
-Louis Pasteur (1822-1895) Scientist
-General George Patton (1885-1945) Military
-Pablo Picasso (1882-1973) Artist
-Edgar Allan Poe (1809-1849) Author, Poet
-Rachmaninov (1873-1943) Composer
-Eddie Rickenbacker (1890-1973) WWI Flying Ace
-John D. Rockefeller (1839-1937) Oil Magnate
-Nelson Rockefeller (1908-1979) U.S. VP
-August Rodin (1840-1917) Artist, Sculptor
-Anna Eleanor Roosevelt (1844-1962) First Lady
-Pete Rose (1941-present) Baseball Player
-Babe Ruth (1895-1948) Baseball Legend
-Nolan Ryan (1947-present) Baseball Player
-Anwar al-Sadat (1918-1981) Egyptian President &
  Nobel Peace Prize Winner in 1976
-George C. Scott (1927-1999) Actor
-George Bernard Shaw (1856-1950) Author
-Will Smith (1968-Present)Actor, Entertainer
-Tom Smothers (1937-present) Actor, Singer

-Socrates (469-399 B.C.) Philosopher (how could they know he had ADD that long ago?)
-Suzanne Somers (1946-present) Actress
-Steven Spielberg (1946-present) Filmmaker
-Sylvester Stallone (1946-present) Actor
-Jackie Stewart (1939-present) Grand Prix Racer
-James Stewart (1908-1997) Actor
-Henry David Thoreau (1817-1862) Author
-Leo Tolstoy (1828-1910) Russian Author (Flunked out of college)
-Alberto Tomba (1966-present) Italian Ski Champ
 -Vincent van Gogh (1853-1890) Artist
-Jules Verne (1828-1905) Author
-Werner von Braun (1912-1977) Rocket Scientist
-Lindsay Wagner (1949-present) Actress
-Robin Williams (1952-present) Comedian
-Woodrow Wilson (1856-1924) U. S. President
-Henry Winkler (1945-present) Actor (Fonzie)
-Stevie Wonder (1950-present) Musician
-F. W. Woolworth (1852-1919) Department Store (While working in a dry goods store at 21, his employers wouldn't let him wait on a customer because he "Didn't have enough sense.")
-Frank Lloyd Wright (1867-1959) Architect
-Orville Wright (1871-1948) Airplane Developer
-Wilber Wright (1867-1912) Airplane Developer
-William Wrigley, Jr. (1933-1999) Chewing Gum Maker
-William Butler Yeats (1865-1939) Irish Author

Note: Names of people with ADD are based on Internet search terms such as "celebrities with ADD" and "famous people with ADD"   see http://www.adhdrelief.com/famous.html

Building on the positive, there are also many strengths in people with ADD. As viewable on Pete Quily's web site:
http://www.addcoach4u.com/positivesofadd.html

Here are 151 positive characteristics of people who have ADHD, which was created in 2003 and it's still one of the most popular pages on his 130 page + website. They include:
- Ability to find alternate paths to overcome obstacles.
- Able to take on large situations.
- Adaptive/collaborative.
- Adventurous, courageous, lives outside of boundaries.
- Always finding alternate routes to any given location.
- Always willing to help others.
- Ambitious – you want to be everything when "you grow up".
- Artistic.
- Attractive personality – magnetic due to high energy.
- Being able to see the big picture.
- Being able to see the patterns in the chaos.
- Being intuitive towards others' difficulties.
- Broad focus – can see more, notice things more.
- Can create order from chaos.
- Can do many projects at once.
- Can make people feel they are heard.
- Can see the big picture.
- Can talk about several things at one time.
- Can think on my feet.
- Career variety.

- Centre of attention.
- Comfortable talking in front of groups.
- Comfortable with change and chaos.
- Compassion for others and for themselves.
- Conceptualizes well.
- Confidence.
- Constantly evolving.
- Courageous.
- Creates connections easily.
- Creative.
- Creative writing.
- Creative – musical, artistic, "dramatic".
- Good in a crisis.
- Good at customer relations.
- Dedicated.
- Detail-oriented.
- Determined to gain more control.
- Eager to make friends.
- Eager to try new things.
- Empathetic, sensitive.
- Energetic.
- Entrepreneurial.
- Excellent organizers using journals and reminders (notes etc.).
- Flexible – changes as the situation requires.
- Fun guy to be around.
- Goal-oriented.
- Good at conceptualizing.
- Good at motivating self and others.
- Good at multitasking.
- Good at problem solving.
- Good at public speaking.
- Good at understanding others/mind reading – empathetic.

- Good conversationalist.
- Good delegator and good at organizing others.
- Good in emergency situations.
- Good listener.
- Good looking and aware of it.
- Good people skills.
- Good self esteem, energetic.
- Great brain-stormer.
- Great multitasker.
- Great self-company.
- Great sense of humor.
- Great storyteller.
- Great with kids (central figure around kids.
- Hands-on workers.
- Hard worker.
- Has friendly relations with their family.
- Has the gift of gab.
- Helpful.
- Helps others who are also in trouble.
- High energy – go, go, go.
- Humor, very healthy, quick picking up ideas.
- Hyperfocus!!
- Hypersensitive – very empathetic and good at non-verbal communications.
- Idea generator.
- Imaginative.
- Impulsive (in a good way) not afraid to act.
- Initiators.
- Intelligent.
- Intuitive.
- It's ok to not finish everything.

- Learning as much as I can to help children and others with ADHD.
- Less sleep is good (midnight to 6 am.)
- Like to talk a lot.
- Likes learning new things.
- Look at multidimensional sides to a situation.
- Lots of interests.
- Loves to cook and be creative.
- Magnetic.
- Master idea generator.
- Mentoring others/helpful.
- Mentoring people with low self esteem.
- Modesty.
- Move on fast – never hold a grudge.
- Multitasks well.
- Never bored and rarely boring.
- Never intimidated to try new things.
- Non-linear, multi-dimensional/edge of chaos.
- Not afraid to speak mind.
- Not contained by boundaries.
- On stage and ready.
- Optimistic.
- Outgoing.
- Passionate.
- Persistent.
- Philosophical.
- Holistic thinking.
- Playful.
- Pragmatic.
- Problem solver.
- Profound.
- Quick thinking.

- Quick witted.
- Relates to people easily.
- Resistant.
- Resourceful.
- See and remember details – recount them later.
- Sees the big picture.
- Socially adaptive and flexible.
- Spontaneous.
- Stabilizer during difficult situations.
- Stable.
- Successful.
- Takes initiative.
- Tenacious.
- Theoretical.
- Think outside the box.
- Thinks 2 meters ahead of the world.
- Thinks big, dreams big.
- Thorough.
- Tolerant.
- Unconventional.
- Unlimited energy.
- Unorthodox.
- Versatile.
- Very creative, able to generate a lot of ideas.
- Very hard working to compensate, workaholic.
- Very intuitive.
- Very resourceful.
- Very successful.
- Visionary.
- Visual learner.
- Willing to explore.
- Willing to take risks.

- Willingness to help others.
- Witty.
- Won't tolerate boredom.
- Works well under pressure.
- Worldly.

A Helpful Tip: Take the paragraph at the beginning of this chapter called Attitude by Charles Swindoll, copy/print it and hang it up somewhere that will allow you to read it every day.

Chapter 2. Symptoms/Behavior

You may be familiar with the typical behavior of individuals with ADD/ADHD. Here is a recap as summarized by The Washington D.C. based American Psychiatric Association; 14 ADD symptoms of Attention Deficit Disorder or ADHD, of which at least eight ADD symptoms of Attention Deficit Disorder of ADHD must be present to be officially classified as Attention Deficit Disorder or ADHD.

SYMPTOMS OF ADD or ADHD:
-Often fidgeting with hands or feet, or squirming while seated.
-Having difficulty remaining seated.
-Being easily distracted by extraneous stimuli.
-Having difficulty awaiting turn in games or group activities.
-Often blurting out answers before questions are completed.
-Having difficulty in following instructions.
-Having difficulty sustaining attention in tasks or play activities.
-Often shifting from one uncompleted task to another.
-Having difficulty playing quietly.
-Often talking excessively.
-Often interrupting or intruding on others.
-Often not listening to what is being said.
-Often forgetting things necessary for tasks or activities.
-Often engaging in physically dangerous activities without considering possible consequences.

The symptoms of ADD are further broken into three specific categories, each with its specific clinical presentation that better describes a child's behavior. These symptoms of ADD categories are Inattentive Type (classic Attention Deficit Disorder), Hyperactive/Impulsive Type (classic Attention Deficit Hyperactive Disorder) and Combined Type (a combination of inattentive and hyperactive).

Inattention symptoms of ADD:

1. Often fails to give close attention to details.
2. Often makes careless mistakes in schoolwork, work, or other activities.
3. Often has difficulty sustaining attention in tasks or play activities.
4. Often becomes easily distracted by irrelevant sights, sounds and extraneous stimuli.
5. Often does not seem to listen when spoken to directly.
6. Often does not follow through on instructions and fails to finish schoolwork, chores, or duties in the workplace.
7. Often has difficulty organizing tasks and activities.
8. Often avoids tasks, such as schoolwork or homework, which require sustained mental effort.
9. Often loses things necessary for tasks or activities, like school assignments, pencils, books, or tools.
10. Often is forgetful in daily activities.
11. Rarely follows instructions carefully and completely.

People with symptoms of ADD who are inattentive display difficulty keeping their mind on any one thing. They may get bored easily with a task and bounce to the next task, and the next task after that. Organizing and completing a task proves troublesome, though they may give undivided and effortless attention to activities and topics they enjoy. People with symptoms of ADD often find that focusing deliberate, conscious attention to learning something new is extremely difficult.

As a result, homework may be agonizing for people with the symptoms of ADD. They might forget to write down assignments or bring home the right books to complete the assignments. When doing homework, people with the symptoms of ADD typically find their minds drifting every few minutes.

Hyperactivity/Impulsive symptoms of ADD:

1. Often fidgets with hands or feet or squirms in seat.
2. Often runs, climbs or leaves seat in settings where remaining seated is expected.
3. Often runs about excessively in situations where it is inappropriate.
4. Often has difficulty playing quietly in leisure activities.
5. Is often "on the go" or often acts as if "driven by a motor."
6. Often talks excessively.
7. Often blurts out answers before hearing the entire question.
8. Often has difficulty waiting turn or for a turn.

9. Often interrupts or intrudes on others at school or work and at home.
10. Often feels and acts restless.

People who display the symptoms of ADD with hyperactivity always seem to be in motion. Sitting still can be an impossible task. They may dash around, squirm in their seats, roam around the room or talk incessantly. They often display repetitive motions like wiggling their feet or tapping their pencil to bring themselves back to focus and burn off excessive energy. Many people who display the symptoms of ADD with hyperactivity feel intensely restless, fidget and may try to do several things at once, bouncing around from one activity to the next.

People who display the symptoms of ADD with impulsivity seem unable to curb their immediate reactions or think before they act. They may blurt out inappropriate comments or run into the street without looking. People with the symptoms of ADD with impulsivity do not "look before leaping." They may grab a toy from another child or hit when they're upset. People who display the symptoms of ADD with impulsivity may find it difficult to wait for things they want or to take their turn in games.

Combined ADHD and ADD symptoms of Attention Deficit Disorder:

1. Includes a mix of symptoms of ADD and ADHD.

A wonderful resource that is also a good first step in the process of diagnosing ADD is the use of an on line screener for symptoms of ADD. A screener by Harvard, NYU & the World Health Organization is located at Pete Quily's web site at www.addcoach4u.com/adultaddtest.html

With so much information available today, such as details of symptoms previously noted and other diagnostic tools, the power to understand, and initiating an action plan against the challenge of ADD can be won.

If only these tools to deal with ADD were available when I was a child, who knows what challenges I could have avoided. Maybe by telling other people about the realities of ADD and countering the stigma and the myths about it, I can make a huge difference in the lives of others with ADD and their families.

However, all of my experiences have made me who I am today. I am fortunate enough to have faced my challenges head-on and turned them into deep personal growth and learning experiences. My behavior earlier in life certainly is easy to recall as I review the list of symptoms. As I scroll down that list, each item brings back memories for me of certain places and times in my life.

I recall fidgeting with my hands or feet, or squirming while seated, only to be told by a teacher to settle down or I'll be sent to detention. I remember sitting in a class room and having great difficulty remaining seated, which also lead to detention time. Ah, such fond memories of the detention room, it was like a second home for me.

Memories of sitting in school and being easily distracted by things like motion in the hall way or activities outside that were visible through the window are still clear in my mind. I was always the class clown, often blurting out answers before questions were completed, usually wrong but I did get the big laughs from my classmates. Maybe I should have been a comedian? Of course like many young children in school, I found myself having difficulty in following instructions as well.

In the past, these symptoms that I displayed were not because I was "poorly disciplined" or "a wild child" or "I needed to grow up". Unfortunately, these challenges I faced were dealt with in detention, being sent to the principals' office or being made an example of in front of my classmates and friends. Fortunately for me, I suffered from an enormous case of narcissism, and self confidence was not a problem. Nothing could beat me down permanently. I was as determined as any person in the world. I may not have achieved "A" grades as a student, but I sure as hell worked hard to pass and subsequently experienced a lot of frustration. It's rather ironic looking back in retrospect that narcissism was such a part of my life as an adult and how it impacted me. It likely was my savior as a child and young boy while growing up in school. I consider myself very fortunate because many children are completely beaten down by their experience with ADD. In fact, it impacts them socially with their circle of friends, peer acceptance and general popularity.

As I grew into an adult, my behavior as an adult also displayed the many symptoms of ADD. The symptoms that I was most challenged by were:

Activating to Work – I was fortunate enough to be organized and come up with a concept or action item, however getting myself to perform that action was always a challenge, procrastinating if you will.

Focusing and Sustaining Focus –I would easily lose track of what I was involved with, including a conversation, work task or listening to someone else.

Processing Speed – I just seemed to be a thought behind everyone else or a little too slow in coming up with a response. This was the biggest challenge for me.

Managing Frustration & Emotions – I was easily frustrated with tasks, actions of others and had a temper. I would soon learn this was directly related to the above mentioned point, Processing Speed.

Narcissism – I had a false sense of who I was and my capabilities.

These traits of ADD defined who I was. I accepted who I was and so did my friends, family, teachers, business associates, girlfriends and wife, now an ex-wife. Unknowingly, I had developed a defense mechanism that allowed me to protect myself with a sharp sense of wit/humor, a way of responding verbally that deflected pressure or others from challenging me. I would regularly give excuses for shortcomings and thereby avoid self-condemnation, disappointment, or criticism by others. I remember hiding my emotional responses and problems under a facade of big words and pretending I had no problem.

I recall a great example of this within the first few years of my working career. I worked in sales and had a boss who would always push me to achieve sales quotas and goals. In retrospect, he was simply doing his job. However, way back then I thought of him as the enemy, not someone who could teach or help me. I remember him putting pressure on me to develop more business, or to increase my sales results. Of course, I had the answers for everything with responses like, "boss, my actions and efforts are what they need to be", or "the market trends are shifting and we need to reestablish how we approach our direct marketing and sales process". This sounded just intelligent enough to get my boss off my back and buy me some more time. Unfortunately, it didn't help me to achieve my goals. Now, this was not the case throughout my career but I can sure recall a couple examples like this.

I would strongly encourage you or anyone you know who could be challenged by ADD to seriously and honestly assess if these or any other symptoms typical of ADD are present. Until a person with ADD can fully understand their symptoms and accept them as reality, that person will not be able to win their battle with ADD.

A Helpful Tip: Try utilizing an online ADD/ADHD screening tool to learn more about

your symptoms, or someone you know at
www.addcoach4u.com and seek professional
medical diagnosis.

Chapter 3. The Wake Up Call

On my 37th birthday, my wife and I stood outside on a beautiful new deck I had built with my own hands in the back yard of our dream home, or so I thought. Funny, I now understand the saying "a house doesn't make a home". To this day I still remember the words exactly as she said them, "I need to leave, I can't do this any more". Those words at that time seemed so surreal, and I was numb. I wasn't numb with pain or hurt as I later discovered, but I was numb with confusion, disorientation and being completely in the dark as to how I had ended up in this situation. ADD had impacted my marriage. There were other issues in my marriage that resulted in its failure as well. However, this is the part of my book where I take the high road. I think it would be easy to list issues and problems that were not my fault in my marriage, however I choose to accept and apologize for my mistakes. I needed to stand up and say "I have ADD" in order to deal with it.

I am a person who has learned and accepted that I am challenged with ADD and it has impacted my life at some point, friends and family negatively. Until I accepted and acknowledged this, I would never be able to work through the challenge. The impact has been apparent with acts of selfishness, being physically and verbally reactive and aggressive. I could not display sympathy or empathy, nor could I feel what it was. I accepted that I was narcissistic, and others viewed me as a narcissist. I believed that this could be limiting me in how others viewed me, related to me or accepted me and in how others viewed me. I had hit that low point in my life, where I was a human being who was not living in reality. Thankfully I was willing to change that. The state that I was in made me incapable of being successful on a long-term basis in a relationship, as a boyfriend, husband, father and friend. This took its toll on me emotionally. I was at the beginning of the end of my marriage with two very young children and I was reeling with confusion and uncertainty. To top it all off, I was living in a community of my wife's choice and was very unhappy there. I was miserable!

I now maneuver differently and am excited about the potential for growth in how I maneuver. I can concentrate more when listening by internally questioning others comments which I never did before. I am more empathetic and sympathetic to others by listening, placing myself in their shoes and trying to feel how they feel.

I am open and willing to do things differently, as I feel I have displayed by seeking counseling and coaching. I feel very confident now that my many challenges and the sources of these challenges have been identified and will be worked on continually.

In regards to how this impacted my life, I became a man who arrived in a much better place. I simply had to prepare myself to be a better man, boyfriend, husband, father and friend by participating in home work exercises, listening, learning to be empathetic and sympathetic, getting a medical diagnosis of ADD, taking meds for ADD etc.. My life started to become more in control regarding my thought process, emotions, reactiveness and general conduct as a person through the above noted activities and continued commitment to making myself better.

In this entire process, I became really affected by how I felt about myself. For some reason I never lost confidence deep down inside myself, but I sure suffered in this growing and learning process. I felt like I had been broken down and was being rebuilt.

Soon, I felt like the light at the end of the tunnel was visible. I gained a true sense of confidence, which was gradually replacing narcissism as a false level of confidence and coping. I am proud of how I accepted my issues and dealt with them. I feel like my future as a man, friend, father and husband (with anyone) will be better and successful. I also feel that I still need to work on myself to ensure my future is successful on all these levels.

A Helpful Tip: Don't be afraid to accept that you have ADD/ADHD and are challenged by it. Accepting this is a powerful step in winning the battle against it.

Chapter 4. Counseling & Medication

One of the first and hardest steps I took was to seek counseling. When I sat in the horribly uncomfortable chair that seemed to have traveled through time via a time machine (dirt included), my mind was closed. It really wasn't very open for a while. As I sat and listened, those typical closed minded thoughts raced through my head like "what a waste of time" and "this guy has read too many self help books".

As time progressed, I derived benefit from the counseling. However, my issues were not being resolved, they were merely covered up by emotional and psychological band aids. In time I came to realize that there was great benefit in counseling, but that this particular counselor was not right for me. In addition, I knew that I was not getting to the root of the challenges with which I was dealing. Off I went in search of the magical and instant cure I was sure existed. A few weeks with a good counselor, I would be on track and normal. Let me tell you, I had a rude awakening when I sat down in the office of Dr. Holly Prochnau, Ph.D. Holly opened my eyes to the reality in which I was living, and it didn't take her long. In just a few sessions, we accomplished more than I had previously accomplished with my first counselor in more sessions than I could count. Thank goodness I made a counseling change, it was for the best and it was the turning point in my progress.

Holly said "Jeff, you have ADD, big time". She was very straightforward and was not afraid to tell me the way it was. There was no beating around the bush with Holly. The hard reality of what was going on in my life had to smack me in the face, and it did. As I sat on yet another old, dirty chair in Holly's office many things went through my mind. The least important, was my curiosity about the possible existence of an association of counselors and psychologists who all purchased bad furniture from the same place. There has to be a market to cash in on here! That is the creative ADD side of me talking :)

All joking aside, Holly and I dove into the many things in my mind and we began to bring the real me to the surface. This was a hard emotional phase in my life. The old saying something along the lines of "you need to hit rock bottom before you can come up again" was very true. I soon realized that I needed to accept the fact that I was challenged by ADD. In my case it had impacted me and was one of the reasons why my marriage failed. I was literally deconstructed in my sessions with Holly, and then reconstructed, in simple terms.

I remember asking Holly her thoughts on where and who I was and where I was going? I don't recall her exact words, but is was along the lines that people don't generally turn it around and I was in a very hard place. She challenged me and told me that this would be a lot of work. I don't know why, how or what happened at that moment, but I took that challenge head-on. Holly's comment made me mad, it had also motivated me. As I walked from Holly's office to my car, I wondered what the hell had happened to my life? I quickly realized in that two minute walk, I needed to turn this ship around and get back on course. I think that my narcissism had placed me in such a place of false self perception, that I unknowingly took that over-confidence and competitiveness within me and said "I am better than this, I am going to win, and nothing is going to stop me"! It was that attitude that propelled me into the hardest period of my life, for the right reasons.

As I continued to work with Holly, one of the major ways we worked was by assigning homework after every session. This homework would be comprised of my answering specific questions in essay and short answers. When I would return with my homework done, there were no gold stars or A's handed out. Instead, we would review the answers I would be sent home to expand further or answer questions that were spawned from the review of my homework. Holly was very good at what she did with me. One assignment we did was really amazing and moving. I had to do a self analysis based on many criteria of my life such as friends, family, career, finances and spirituality. This was an exercise that created a tremendous amount of work for me, and as it was nearing the completion stage Holly asked me to do another assignment. Instead of self analysis, she asked me to have a friend write me an honest letter about who I am and review some strengths and weaknesses. I called on a good friend of mine, and here are his words:

"Jeff,
Further to our discussion earlier in the week, you had asked that I put some thoughts down on paper in regards to my thoughts of the type of person I perceive you as and the way that I have seen you over the years of our friendship.

To start off, how can I not thank you for the GREAT friend you have been to me personally, and to the others in my family. There have been many occasions in the past where I had needed a friend to talk to and to understand and help me through some difficult personal times. You were always there for me even if it might not have been the best timing for you.

When I was going through a divorce in 1998, I always knew that if I needed someone to talk to or to bounce some thoughts off, you were always there with some helpful insight and support. There are so many reasons, too many to number why I consider you one of my closest friends.

Over the 17 or so years that we have been friends we have been through it all with each other. Starting as friends at University , coworkers in the restaurant business, roommates after I graduated and the list goes on.

After I moved to the West coast, our friendship remained strong. It was obvious from the way you worked to keep our friendship on track by calling and visiting on a regular basis that you were committed to maintaining our friendship. Whenever we got together it was as if things had never changed, as if we were still roommates.

Our careers over the past ten years have taken different directions. New and exciting fields for both of us, but you have always shown interest and understanding as to why I chose the field and direction that I did. I have always appreciated the support.

We have partnered on boat ownership/racing and been through-many close calls on the water (tight mark roundings) and other high anxiety situations. We have always managed to never walk away too pissed off and have always managed to put it behind us and carry on the following day, knowing that things were all good. Well, there was the odd occasion where we had to sit down and work it through to ensure that things ran smoothly on the boat, but never was our friendship in jeopardy. As we both know, sailing/racing has been the end of many friendships and even some marriages.

As time moves on and friendships evolve and change, I have seen a whole new side of you. Your marriage has always seemed like a great partnership to me. The way the two of you were able to move around, doing chores and running a household always appeared for the most part effortless. You both seemed to share jobs/chores around the house without conflict.

Your ability to entertain my son when I came over was awesome. He still thinks of you as my coolest friend. (God only knows why!) He's only 9. He'll come to his senses soon! I knew by the way you reacted with him that you too would one day be a great father.

As I watch your kids grow and I see how you react and handle raising them I commend you on your hard work and patience with them. You are calm, level headed and always take the time to explain and teach them and challenge them to think instead of taking the easy route and reprimanding and/or raising your voice. I know with your continued hard work with them they will be great kids and young adults in the not too distant future.

On many occasions when our families have gotten together and I end up sitting and chatting with your wife she had always nothing but great things to say to me about your ability as a father and how people should be lucky to have you as a friend. On that note I must say that this is a letter that could be written by a dozen people across this country who would consider you as close a friend as I do.

You are a great friend and I hope with all my heart that things will work out and that you and your wife can get things back on track and moving forward. With the commitment and resolve that I know you have, I have great confidence that if it is possible, you will do what is required to make it work. Here are your STRENGTHS AND WEAKNESSES AS I SEE THEM:

AS A FRIEND, PERSON, FATHER AND HUSBAND
<u>*Strengths*</u>
- *Loyal*
- *Outgoing*
- *Thoughtful*
- *Caring*
- *Patient with his children*
- *Willing to do his fair share of household duties*
- *Friendly*
- *Warm and welcoming of new people*
- *Jeff is working on being more open minded and listening to input from others*

- *Open to the idea that he is not always perfect, and is interested in improving areas of weakness*

Weaknesses

- *Sees his opinion as the right one in financial decisions and assumes that his wife will eventually come to understand and agree with his decision*

- *Sometimes makes quick decisions without working through both positive and negative, and considering the alternatives*

- *Can be frivolous with money at times*

- *In the past, when he has set his mind on something, it is almost impossible to present another option to him.*
- *Doesn't back-check while playing hockey"*

Wow, was I ever moved after reading that letter. My friend's letter was a real eye opener, he confirmed my actions which related to ADD, but he also let me know I was a decent guy, who needed some improvement and help. I have a tremendous amount of respect for my friend who wrote this letter, because he was honest enough to speak his mind. I'm not sure if he realized how much this letter impacted me and meant to me? Well, he does now!

As this process was continuing, my wait for an appointment with Dr. Gabor Mate had finally arrived. Vancouver based Dr. Mate and author of *Scattered Minds* is recognized as an accomplished specialist in ADD and he did confirm/diagnose that I was challenged by ADD. I was required to complete a questionnaire prior to attending my assessment appointment, as was my x-wife. The two completed questionnaires along with other diagnosis tools would offer Dr. Mate a good perspective of me, as I saw myself and as another saw me. Once the diagnosis was complete, I took some time to consider some medication options that Dr. Mate had recommended. I came to the conclusion that Concerta would be the best choice for me.

After meeting with Dr. Mate once again, he wrote me a prescription and I commenced my Concerta stage. When I asked Dr. Mate how long it would take to notice the effect of the medication, he said "within 24-48 hours". I was very surprised as I expected a much longer time frame. He was also quick to point out that the medication would not correct the challenges that I faced with ADD. In simple terms, the medication would allow the circuits in my brain to start firing back and forth. Once these circuits were firing, my brain would be in a state capable of learning, retaining and correcting it's self. Both Dr. Mate and Holly were very clear that medication alone was not the answer, I would also need to dedicate myself to learning life skills and alternate ways of feeling and thinking.

Both Dr. Mate and Dr. Hallowell have both stated, "pills don't teach skills", it takes more than that. Dr. Mate was very accurate in his estimate of how long it would take for the medication to kick in. About 30 hours into the meds it hit me like you could not imagine! It was as if those brain circuits that were not firing previously, suddenly came alive and absolutely knocked me sideways. It was as if I suddenly came out of a fog. I felt emotions that I had never felt, and understood things I had never understood. I went through a two week period where my brain was processing all the emotions and thoughts it should have been processing over many years. I was an emotional wreck as I experienced emotions like never before. One of the biggest impacts I experienced was my ability to understand, how to feel empathetic and sympathetic, which is detailed in Chapter 11.

I soon came to a point in the counseling process with Holly where I felt that I needed more. The progress I experienced with Holly was valuable and I am very grateful for everything she helped me with. After my progress and hard work to that point, I knew there was a lot more work to do still. That work would be accomplished by learning life skills and seeking counseling with an ADD specific person, a coach.

A Helpful Tip: Through counseling, I realized the strength my family and friends were capable of providing me. Lean on your family and friends, they are here to help.

Chapter 5. Coaching

Enter Pete Quily. Pete is an Adult ADHD and life skills coach. Pete started by letting me know that coaching works best when you have clear goals, which are based on your needs and values. "We will work together to refine your goals", said Pete.

The ability to reflect back, or hindsight as it is commonly referred to is cruel, I always thought. Why couldn't we have the ability to do the exact opposite, use foresight. A light went on inside my mind and I realized that the lessons and skills I was learning were starting to allow me to think differently and as a result, I started seeing potential situations differently, feeling differently and visualizing potential outcomes through my new thought process, a little foresight, if you will.

I look back on the past years of this experience and I see two points in my life where I turned a corner, for the better. One corner I turned was when my wife left me. Although I did not realize it at the time, it was a wonderful gift that set me free, thanks Shannon! The other corner I turned was with Pete Quily. Maybe it was a culmination of events, efforts, pain, growth and learning that brought me to this point. It's possible a little miracle may have occurred or maybe, just maybe, two paths on a journey in life crossed and it was just meant to be. No matter what the reasons were that I turned that corner in life, Pete Quily and I turned that corner together forever changing my life.

Openly and publicly I say to you Pete, thank you for saving my life. Not in sense of life and death, but in relation to my life progressing positively instead of moving in a negative direction.

My first coaching session, Pete and I met by phone. That's how Pete does it, and for me it was very effective. We chatted about my journey through ADD, what I had experienced and where I was going. We learned about each other and agreed that we would start regular phone coaching sessions. Three times a month Pete and I scheduled a time to talk for 30 minutes. Regularly, our time would run well beyond the allotted time. Generously and without doubt, Pete would always let our sessions continue past the allotted time. Prior to each session, I would have to complete Pete's coaching prep form and email it to him so that he could prepare for the session. Pete's form asked that I fill in the follow statements:

1. This week I am grateful for -
2. The commitments that I made to myself on our last call were -
3. What I was able to do around those commitments included
4. What I did not get done that I had intended to
5. What challenges am I facing right now, and how am I handling them?
6. What opportunities are available to me now?
7. I have made new insights and realizations?
8. Any changes I would like to see in our relationship or the coaching process?
9. Something that would make our coaching session more effective, useful or fun?
10. What do I want to focus on in my next call

At the end of every coaching session, we had created a list of goals to accomplish for the next coaching session. These goals varied greatly and included:

a) Use of catch phrases
b) Relationship interactions
c) Rewards
d) Trying new things
e) Parenting
f) Communicating
g) Thought processes
h) Emotional levity

I've borrowed some content from his web site www.addcoach4u.com as I feel it can be of benefit to people who may need the coaching that I was fortunate enough to receive. Working with a sensitive and empathic coach is a healthy way to grow. Most clients hire a coach to accomplish several specific goals and much of the time may be spent working on these goals. Yet, with coaching, don't be surprised if you discover new parts of yourself or if you find your goals adjusting themselves to who you really are. This discovery process is natural, so you needn't rush it, just realize it will likely happen.

Accelerated personal and professional growth is the hallmark of being coached. Part of working with Pete as your coach is that he will ask a lot of you, not too much, but certainly more than you have likely been asked before. You will experiment with fresh approaches and must be open to redesigning parts of your life to your best ability. This is so you

can more easily reach your goals and live an
integrated and fulfilled personal and professional
life, using your gifts and enjoying life as it was
meant to be enjoyed. Your homework will be tasks,
actions and resulting results or shifts in your
behavior. You do the best you can to accomplish
these tasks before your next phone call. You must
apply yourself and use the homework to help you
achieve your personal and professional goals.

It is helpful if you purchase a note pad to make
notes in during your calls, to track progress or write
thoughts and reflections in. Your gremlin is your
inner critic, evil twin, and when he/she catches a
whiff of significant life change, it's likely to show
up with lots of reasons why this program shouldn't
go one step farther. "This is stupid, you're not
ready, I have never been able to do this before, I am
not good enough, etc." His job is to keep you
where you are. Just because you have come to Pete
to help make significant changes in your life, your
gremlin will not disappear immediately. Be willing
to tackle your inner critic/gremlin!

Once you have made a commitment to coaching
and to change, you have a lot invested in success.
The first time you meet disappointment, the first
time your outcome eludes your grasp, you may
think the whole plan has collapsed. Look rather at
this as an outcome with an opportunity to learn.

Expect ups and downs, plateaus, periods of great
insight, everything happening at lightning speed,
followed by the wake of the wave, drifting in the
doldrums. For most clients there's a slump between
weeks three and eight. Change is not happening fast

enough and your initial euphoria of commitment has worn off.

There may be times when Pete may ask for permission to tell you what he thinks. For example: "may we brainstorm an alternative course of action?"

Pete is likely to intrude in the middle of your story to ask a directed question. He may rigorously challenge your thinking. This intrusion might be considered rude in polite social conversation, but is a powerful aspect of your coaching conversation, designed to cut to the heart of the matter.

If you or someone you know may require an ADHD coach, I can say that it was a very successful process for me. I would urge anyone considering coaching to further investigate this process, it just may be a turning point in your life or someone you know. For me, it was the required next step after starting my medication phase and I know that it was a required piece of my puzzle. The coaching process is indeed proof that, **pills don't teach skills**.

One of the most effective coaching wins I experienced with Pete was the implementation of a little exercise called "take a step back". No matter what the circumstance was, if I ever found myself in a situation that required deep thought, a response in a volatile or heated situation or control of my emotions, I trained my brain to automatically think "take a step back". This would allow me the extra second to hold back on responding in certain situations, think at a deeper level and respond or communicate in a more effective and appealing way. The results were noticeable and very pleasing. I listened, spoke and thought like a different person. Coaching for me, was the key factor in winning my challenges against ADD.

I feel that the biggest reason coaching worked for me was because it offered a non-biased sounding board that is not personally linked to me, my family or friends. A qualified and experienced Coach keeps the best interests of his or her client in mind.

A Helpful Tip: Get an ADD/ADHD coach. Don't procrastinate or over think it, just do it! It changed my life.

Chapter 6. Meds Are Not Enough

The phrase "pills don't teach skills" is one of the most accurate and impacting statements I heard during my period of work dealing with ADD. It took a while for me to understand and truly grasp the impact of this statement. I read it, I heard it from two doctors and my ADD coach.

So, what exactly did I need to do? I needed to completely understand my challenges, how they impacted me and how to overcome them. There were two steps I would need to take in order to overcome my challenges:

- start medication
- learning and maintaining new life skills.

Taking medication, that was the easy part. I did very well with that, the pill went in my mouth and down it went with a quick sip of water. Joking aside, that was just the beginning and the medication allowed my brain to be ready to learn and retain new skills. This is of course a simplified description of what occurred.

Once I started my medication, I began the hardest part of my learning, I became consumed by coaching, books, internet research, practicing new skills and dedicating myself to beating ADD. I opened up to as many possible ways to beat ADD as I could wrap my arms around. Unfortunately, many people will resist looking inward. I had to come up with the courage to look at myself on the inside, and improve how I reacted outside my body and mind. Here is what I focused on over an intense two year period and continue with today:

Self Awareness – In many ways this was one of the most emotionally upsetting steps of growing. By becoming aware of myself and my challenges, I had to take a very serious look at me in the mirror and realize who I was and more importantly, accept it. Realizing what my weaknesses and challenges were left me feeling very vulnerable and inadequate. However, this was the most important step in the first of many steps that would lead to my victory. My commencement of counseling with Dr. Holly Prochnau forced me to start the process of understanding who I was.

Coaching – ADD coaching was the hinge pin that held my entire learning process together. It was intense, relaxing, upsetting, rewarding and incredibly thought provoking. It seemed like an emotional roller coaster in the beginning. As time progressed it became less of a roller coaster and I began to see, feel and realized real results. Letting go of my inhibitions regarding coaching and really opening up was an important factor in my coaching sessions becoming effective and successful.

Books – Never having been much of a reader as a result of having ADD, I found myself starting to enjoy reading for the first time in my life. I started slowly by limiting the amount of time I would read. I eventually increased the time and made sure I was in the right environment where I could relax and concentrate. I recall finishing a couple books in their entirety in all the years of my life, but now I was finishing books and enjoying it. The first two books I read were *Scattered Minds* by Dr. Gabor Mate and *The Laws of The Spirit* by Dan Millman. Both books proved to be informative, educational and enjoyable.

Listening – Typically I would talk too much and never take the time to listen to others, as well as interrupt people when they were speaking. This had to change and I needed to listen more before talking. A funny thing happened when I shut my mouth and open my ears, I actually started hearing things differently. Others had the chance to finish what they were saying and the message I received was complete. This made a huge difference in how I interacted with others. I practiced this in conversations with friends, business associates and family. I initially had to bite my tongue, however the process of teaching myself to listen became easier and resulted in a wonderful way of communicating more effectively.

Speaking – The tone you speak in can send the wrong message and ultimately, that impacts how you or what you are saying is perceived. I needed to reinvent the tone of my communication. I actually started recording my phone conversations, both in business and personally. I was amazed how I sounded and realized that there was some improving to do. Recording my calls really made me aware of tone and how important it was. Hearing myself allowed me to think about how important the tone I spoke in was and by improving this, I started to see people respond more positively when I spoke.

Relationships – I received a lot of support from my friends and family, I was and am very fortunate to have some very strong relationships. One day I woke up and realized that any relationship worth keeping was a lot of work. I needed to work harder on some of my relationships, with many of the items that you are reading about right now in this chapter. However, I also noticed that there were relationships in my life where the other individual was not giving back anything. In these cases, I was clearly the initiator when it came to picking up a phone to say hi, visiting or sending an email. I decided to test these relationships and stopped communicating with some people to see what happened. Of the many relationships I am fortunate enough to have, only two ended. All the relationships I still had were strengthened by my actions towards improving myself and by my test or experiment. While this test may or may not be something you do, please be sure to use the support of your friends and family.

Thinking – How I thought really was transformed in this huge learning process. However, I can look at two simple lessons I learned about thinking and that dramatically impacted me and I still use. The first was learning to, take a step back. I actually scheduled the message "take a step back" into my daily Outlook calendar so that it would notify me a few times a day, including on my Blackberry when I was away from my computer. When that notification reminder pops up on my computer or on my Blackberry, I stop what I'm doing and take a moment to reflect on how my day is going and what I can improve on. The second process that was very beneficial was learning to ask myself, "what's the story in my head?"

Occasionally I would over-think myself into a problem. As an example, if my boss sent me an email asking to set up a time to speak with me, I would start thinking too much about it and create a false perception of the pending call. Now, I simply ask myself "what's the story in my head?" By doing this, I answer the question with more positive results.

Managing Stress – This is such an important factor in the improved quality of my life. For each person managing stress can be accomplished in many ways. For me, stress was dramatically reduced by exercise and learning to relax a little bit more. I can not emphasize this point enough to people who are challenged by ADD. You must discover what your outlet is for relieving stress. I also found listening to relaxation CD's or linking to relaxation web sites to be very effective as well.

Relaxing – Taking time to relax was never my strong point. I thought relaxing was flopping down on the couch after a long day and continually changing channels on the TV with the remote. I realized through coaching that I needed to schedule time to relax, before I was exhausted. On a work day, I schedule a ten minute break to sit and have a cup of tea in the middle of my work day. I like going to the beach for a sunset or listening to some relaxing music, these are just a few ways I've learned to relax.

Working – my ability to work has improved dramatically with one skill that I was very poor at previously, reprioritizing. I was great at setting my list of goals or to-do's. However, in the busy pace of a work day I needed to regularly reprioritize and I failed to work effectively as a result. Today, I actually schedule two reprioritizing points during my work day and this has offered me a very positive improvement in my work day.

Children – Wow, I could write an entire book on just this topic. In summary, with the areas of improvement I needed to work on, it all rolled up into being a better father to my children. I believe I always was a good father but like so much in life, there is always room for improvement. The level of patience I displayed, the stress of parenting, teaching and being a stable influence are all areas that I focused on.

After focusing on all these areas of self improvement intensely for years in combination with medication, I started to see and feel results. Many of the things that challenged me no longer did or the impact was lessened. I finally felt like all of my work and efforts were being rewarded. The amount of effort, time and dedication I channeled in to working through ADD had paid off and I understood the often heard phrase, "pills don't teach skills".

A Helpful Tip: If you chose to utilize medication, investigate and ask questions to ensure you make an informed and educated decision regarding what is best for you. Make sure your doctor or psychiatrist really knows ADD, many have not been trained in diagnosing and treating ADD.

Chapter 7. When Has Medication Done Its Job?

The benefits of medication can not be argued in my case. They were an important part of the puzzle in winning my battle against ADD. There also comes a certain point in time for some people, not necessarily all people, but in my case, to stop taking medication. The medication had done its job. *Please seek professional medical advice regarding any decisions you make pertaining to the use of medication.*

I was on Concerta for just under two years and as noted by Dr. Gabor Mate when I originally started, there was and is no way to know how long I would be required to be on medication. There are people who have been on medication for years and years, some for a short period of time and some who will never be able to leave medication alone. For me and fortunately, I experienced success with medication and the time came for me to reevaluate its use. One of the experiences I went through on medication was an incredible awakening of self. As I progressed with learning and personal growth, it was very clear in my circumstance that the medication was an effective and useful tool in winning this challenge. During this process I always had that underlying thought of getting off the medication one day. When that day would be, I had no idea. When I started the medication and continued with the personal work, I noticed that there was a big difference in how I processed a situation, thought and reacted. The medication gave me that extra split second I needed to react properly. As time passed this split second and my thought process and reaction started to become second nature. The events that would normally have frustrated me started to become events that I would deal with correctly. I was winning the battle and that felt great! After a visit with my family doctor, we determined that I would try to start the process of slowly weaning myself off of the medication. I had decided to start investigating this based on some occurrences that drew me to the conclusion that, I just may have progressed past the benefits of medication. I may have arrived at that place where, it was now up to me to be who and what I was capable of being.

The weaning off medication started and I found that in general it was a successful process. My weaning off process was slow and drawn out over a period of time. I took one pill every other day during this process. Initially I noticed that on the days when I took a pill, I seemed a little more together and benefited from the medication. On the days when I would not take a pill, I noticed that I would be somewhat challenged at times with the issues that challenged me in the past. However, these issues that challenged me previously did not challenge me to the point of frustration and confusion that they once did. These issues challenged me to react, think, perceive and generally deal with them in a new way that I had learned.

My brain had gone through the process of the circuits firing or creating new neural pathways and my brain had absorbed new lessons and experiences. These life skills that I had dedicated myself to learning and becoming second nature had started to work. I was very excited! Towards the end of weaning off of my medication I started to notice that there was a swing in my behavior, thoughts and emotions. On the days when I took a pill, I was more emotional and reactive than on the days when I did not take a pill. I believe that since the medication I was on is also a stimulant, I had reached a point in the process where I was becoming over stimulated. My brain and its capabilities had caught up to the benefits of the medication, in simple terms.

After discussions with my family doctor and ADD coach, I decided it was time to stop taking medication. I was about to leave on vacation for a 10 day Spring get away into the warm sun shine. This was perfect timing and I would use this opportunity to do a tremendous amount of self anyalization and reflection. During my vacation I soaked up the sun down south with my folks in Florida. During the visit I would do a self evaluation of events, conversations and thoughts I had experienced. As an example, if I were in a conversation with my Dad I would review my words, how I expressed myself and how I perceived his words in that conversation. You could say that I went through a review of everything I did on numerous occasions in a day.

Upon reviewing these pieces of my day, I came to a few conclusions. The most prominent conclusion was that I had indeed hit a point where I felt confident in stopping my medication. I had learned, I had grown and I had become a better man. However, this was not the end, it was just another step along the way to overcoming ADD.

I now started experiencing a period of second guessing myself. With my not taking medication any more, I realized that I was now on my own. It was time to think, feel and react to everything on my own. We are all human and to error is human. Everyone will make mistakes and perhaps wish they could do something over again, differently.

I was experiencing everything in life that you could imagine and on occasion I found myself wondering, if I reacted a certain way, was it because I was simply human and made mistakes everyone makes or because I had ADD? I soon realized that I was human and that I could not beat myself up emotionally or psychologically every time I reacted, thought or spoke. I needed to take a step back and realize that I had accomplished a tremendous amount in the time I had been working on myself and that as long as I continued to be aware of the fact that I was challenged by ADD and continued to work on myself, I was being the best person I could.

After an extended period of time of being off the medication, I had gained confidence in my ability to think, react and communicate naturally and on my own. The challenge I faced now was not unlike a golfer trying to maintain his game and skills or a business executive growing by staying on top of the latest market trends. I needed to solidify my skills, build on them and continue to learn and grow as a person. I could not stand still just because I had achieved success. I believe everyone should think this way, whether they have ADD or not. It can only make you a better person.

After so much growth, I certainly was mentally and emotionally exhausted. Knowing that I had to continue to evolve and grow, I decided to take a break and give myself a mental and emotional holiday. This was exactly what I needed. I set a scheduled date in advance noting when my internal vacation would be over and when that day arrived, I would start the personal growth process once again.

During my internal vacation, I went through some periods where I was able to reflect back and proudly recognized my accomplishments and actions. I also was aware of certain things that could be improved upon. During this process, I really dove into the writing of this book. While writing I experienced something I had not counted on, the process of writing turned into an enjoyable experience and allowed me to summarize what I had been through, where I was going and provided closure to many issues. It was a great experience!

A Helpful Tip: Track your behavior changes before and during taking medication, in a log of activity results. It is important to gauge your progress and make informed decisions regarding medication and other actions to win a battle against ADD.

Chapter 8. Power of The Mind

Have you ever been formally introduced to your best friend and your worst enemy at the same time? Let me introduce you to your mind.

Your mind has so much capability of creating an incredible life that will offer you back experiences and gifts you could not even dream of. There is one catch to this however, we need to find a way to remain in control of our minds in order to accomplish this. If we lose control, the mind will race out of control. We have the capability to impact the direction our minds go or function in. If we don't manage that direction, the mind will eventually run amok, and that is when you will come face to face with your worst enemy. Thank goodness we have the capability to learn and lead a great life, if we chose to. Unfortunately how to live a rewarding and great life is not a standard text book we get in school and it is a never ending learning process we all need to take on. According to Chuck Gallozzi at Personaldevelopment.com which can be seen at the following link http://www.personal-development.com/chuck/yourmind.htm our life unfolds, for better or worse, as our mind goes through the following three steps.

1) Things stimulate our senses and create thoughts in our conscious mind.

2) The thoughts are sent to our subconscious mind where they become beliefs.

3) The beliefs are automatically acted on, resulting in either negative or positive behavior.

In Chuck Gallozzi's writings, he refers to an experience where we have all probably heard parents say to their children things like "why are you so clumsy? You're always bumping into things!" I love this example, it really serves as a real life situation that parents can all relate to, or allows adults to reflect back on things that were said to them growing up. If the child hears this type of comment, the thought is created. Then that thought becomes a belief and the child's beliefs are then acted on.

We need to be very careful of what we say, our words have impact and shape how our minds develop.

When our brains take that comment about always being clumsy or bumping into things, our subconscious creates many feelings.

Now, my untrained medical opinion tells me the thoughts in our mind have to be converted into a visual image like a picture before they become part of our subconscious. Once again I love the example Chuck Gallozzi uses, about the parent and the clumsy child. "Don't bump into the coffee table!" the parent shouts at her child. "I mustn't bump into the table" thinks the child.

Our message and our words need to focus on the positive message instead. We know how powerful our words can be, so imagine programming a positive and empowering message in the mid of a person you are speaking to.

When my son played little league baseball, myself and the other parents did not stand on the side lines yelling at the kids messages like "don't miss the ball" or "don't strike out". There is always one parent who says things that are a little shocking though. Instead, we offered messages of encouragement and empowerment to the kids that sounded like "hit the ball" or "you can do it" or "have fun" or when they struck out "great job" or "good try, that was a great swing".

This messaging is about focusing on the behavior and positivity we want. I like the simplicity of what Chuck Gallozzi said, "hit the ball" easily translates into a picture. However, this is not the case for, "don't miss the ball!"

We have all heard the sayings like "the power of positive thought" or "have a good attitude". I have learned that repeating this thought process or saying positive things embeds them into my subconscious or my kid's subconscious. I carry a better attitude and disposition forward and I can see the determination and confidence in my kids when they are trying to accomplish something.

If you think and speak positively, good things will usually happen to you and the people around you. If you think negatively or speak negative thoughts, it's pretty easy to guess what kind of results you will get and how others around you will be impacted, right?

Within our thoughts and subconscious it is also important to set goals. I have touched on goals in a previous chapter and our goals tie directly into a positive attitude, mind-set and subconscious. If I set a goal of being in better shape in six months and in six months I can do five more push-ups, that's great. What if I can do five more push-ups in six months but I've gained 15 pounds of fat? My goal needs to be specific and the baby steps or actions that result in a goal needs to be detailed. Instead, my goal might be better if I set out to be in better shape in six months by doing ten more push-ups every day, walking fifteen minutes every day and designing a healthier food and nutrition plan.

In my case, my thoughts have evolved into repetition and that repetition has helped me create habits that impact the state of my mind in a very positive way. Henry David Thoreau said in simpler terms: "Thought is the sculptor who can create the person you want to be. I start using my thought-chisels to become the person I was meant to be."

When we are focused, we do not waste our time or energy. If I am organized, have a plan and have created a road map regarding when and how I will execute my plan, I am very productive and I am utilizing the power of my mind.

My powerful mind is also more capable when I exercise regularly. I have found that I could always find the time to exercise each day, no matter how busy I was. If I could do that, you can too. Forget all your excuses like you do not have the time, or you are too busy. Unless you are prevented from exercise by a medical or physical impairment, no excuses please, find a place and way to exercise in a way that is right for you. This commitment will improve the power of your mind and make it easier to concentrate.

Concentration was always hard for me when I was younger. I remember when I was in college and I needed to study for an exam. I sat comfortably on the couch with the book in my hands and started reading. After a while I felt hungry and went to the kitchen to eat something. I returned to read, and then heard people talking outside. I listened to them for several moments and then brought my attention back to the book. When distractions interfered I felt restless and switched on the radio to listen to some music or watched music videos on TV. I continued to read for a little while, and then remembered something that happened the day before, and then I started thinking about it.

When I looked at my watch, I was amazed to find out that one complete hour had passed and I had hardly read anything!

If you have ADD like me, this scenario likely conjures up feelings of familiarity. There are many situations in life, where a little concentration can make a great difference. Find out where or when you could use more concentration. Imagine what you could have accomplished, if you possessed better concentration. Our minds are powerful, we can end up very happy or very unhappy. We are in control, it is up to us to make ourselves happy.

A Helpful Tip: Look deeply and honestly inside yourself and ask, what do I need to improve on to start winning the challenge against ADD? Try some meditation and concentration exercises. Set realistic goals, no matter what goal you choose and the actions you plan to achieve this.

Chapter 9. The Brain's Capability

With ADD, the challenges I faced are simply explained by stating; certain circuits in my brain did not develop properly. However, those circuits existed, they just needed to start firing. Once the circuits started to fire, my brain had the ability to learn, retain and overcome this challenge.

I found many books very informative and useful in trying to understand ADD, my brain and how they related. In Dr. Gabor Mate's book Scattered Minds, he was very clear in explaining the two following points:

- ADD is not an inherited illness, but a reversible impairment, a developmental delay
- With ADD, circuits in the brain whose job is emotional self-regulation and attention control fail to develop in infancy

At this point in time, I realized that my brain was going to be an important factor in working through ADD. In addition, I learned that ADD was not a disease, it was as Dr. Mate had stated, "a reversible impairment or a developmental delay."

I became filled with confidence because I knew that I could win my battle against ADD. I have battled against many obstacles that I thought were insurmountable in my life and won those battles. I knew that I could do this. I knew that I could harness the capability of my brain.

Today modern medical findings via advanced neurological research have shown us that a challenge such as ADD is more than just a condition of heredity. Today, we now know that the causes of ADD can also be attributed to the social and psychological conditions that shape the brains of children. As noted by Dr. Gabor Mate: "We now know that the anatomy of the brain, the shape and configuration of the myriads of circuits that make up the brain's apparatus is not set by heredity alone, but by also the environment. Environment, too, helps to determine the chemistry of the brain."

The amazing thing about our human brain, is that it's development is limitless. We don't even know what the limitations of the human brain are! As our brain development begins outside the uterus, we are subject to such an incredible amount of influence by so many sources, it is really not surprising that our brains have such potential for development on a continual basis throughout life.

Our brain circuit development goes through a survival and growth process that has been referred to as "Neural Darwinism". Basically, brain circuits that experience stimulation grow and start firing or working as they should. However with ADD, there are some brain circuits that fail to develop and grow. An example of this would be plugging the nose of a young child for many years in their early stages of development. That child would not smell, therefore it would not develop the brain circuits associated with that task, or sense.

So this leads to the question: what is going wrong with the development or growth of a person's brain which results in the condition of ADD?

According to Dr. Gabor Mate:

"In attention deficit disorder the chief physiological problem appears to be located in the frontal lobe of the brain, in the area of the cortex (or gray matter) where attention is allocated and emotions and impulses are regulated. Just as the visual circuits need the stimulation of light, the circuits of attention and emotion control also need the appropriate input: a calm, non-stressed connection with a non-stressed and non-distracted primary maternal caregiver. Stresses on the mothering adult-or disruption of contact with her, as in adoption-predispose children to ADD because they directly affect the developing electrical circuits of the infant's brain. The very chemistry of the infant's brain is affected."

It is true the frontal lobes are a big part of ADD, says Pete Quily, but they're not the only part. There's also the temporal lobes, caudate nucleus, anterior cingulated etc.. See some of the research here at http://addcoach4u.com/doesaddreallyexist.html#cli nicalevidenceoftheexistenceofadd

It is clear now that the parenting environment in the first five years of a child's life does impact the development of the child's brain. This is not to say that an adult such as myself who has ADD experienced a horrible upbringing and parental environment. My parents did the best they could at that place in time. However, the environment that is created by parents or a parent, will impact the child's brain development. I feel that most parents likely do the best that they can with the knowledge that they have. Today, the knowledge that is at our disposal is almost limitless. Whether on the Internet, via books like those by Dr. Mate, Dr. Amen or Dr. Hallowell, so much information and knowledge to help our society develop the brains of our young exists today. Please take advantage of these resources.

Part of the ADD mystery is linked to the challenging social factors that parents face in our society today. The traditional family that once was the majority in North America has been replaced by a new definition of family that includes step parents, step siblings, single fathers, single mothers and shared custody situations. The development of children's brains is usually not the concern of most parents. What is most concerning, is the stress that is placed on the parents and children in these environments. I know this first hand from when my parents divorced and when I experienced a divorce as well. Stress is caused by family breakdowns, work, relationship strain and the general hectic pace of life we live today.

We now know that the brains circuits can still develop new capabilities or the ability to fire later in life. In my experience, the success I have achieved regarding my brain circuit development of new capabilities or the ability to fire, has been achieved through a long-term healing goal which included medications, ADD coaching, life skills coaching, reading, research and my very dedicated effort to self improvement. Until I was diagnosed with ADD, I understood this disorder about as well as the average North American doctor, which is to say hardly at all. Today, ADD/ADHD is still a minor component of most medical training programs. For example, a student at UBC medical school in Vancouver BC only gets about one hour of training on ADHD.

I am not a doctor, so please keep this in mind as I am not offering medical advice. For me, I need to challenge my brain, get out of ruts. It seems to be obvious through my experience and it is medically supported, that simply changing habits and environment stimulates the brain enough to create new connections. Little things like switching the side of the bed you sleep on, changing your daily routine or reading something upside down can accomplish this. Don't be afraid of trying something different or doing something different.

I have a good friend whom I do road trips with from Vancouver to Seattle. We'll drive south for a couple hours to go see a baseball game, have a few beers and check the city out. Whenever I have been to Seattle in the past, I tended to gravitate to the same restaurant, the same bar, the same tourist trap and the same hotel. As we were driving down recently on I-5, I said to my friend that he was in control of all social decisions for the weekend, I was in his hands. My thought was that this would force me into a place in which I would experience new things, experiencing new senses, thoughts and emotions. Also, it would break that routine of repetition that I had fallen into. That decision was so important in my dealing with ADD. Something so simple, yet so moving. That weekend getaway was a fantastic time! My good friend provided me a whole new Seattle experience. I ate at restaurants I never knew existed. I discovered the best serving of scallops I have ever had in my life! The scenery was suddenly different as I let him decide what left and right turns to make. I saw buildings and architecture that I had never noticed before. Unfortunately, the Seahawks absolutely blew it against the Rams when we attended the football game, but hey, I didn't expect a total miracle! All of a sudden my brain was coming even more alive by breaking the normal routine.

It is also proven scientifically that the importance of a proper diet impacts how your brain functions. Brain conscious food includes low saturated fats and eating fatty fish, greens, fruit and nuts. Your brain needs food, blood, oxygen and stimulation. The brain is the most incredible organ in your body. Think about it, of all your organs the brain is the only one that can't really be transplanted. If your brain is removed, your mind, thoughts, subconscious, feeling and every memory and emotion you have ever experience is gone. It controls your body's temperature, blood pressure, heart rate, and breathing. The brain looks after all the motions your body does automatically, like walking, running, and reaching for things, without you having to think about how to do it. The brain does all of these things faster and more effectively than the most powerful computer we have ever seen, yet it is only slightly bigger than the size of two of my adult fists. The brain makes up only about 2% of your body weight, and consumes 25%

of the blood from every heart beat, thus activities that help the heart also help the brain.

Brain 101 – Your Mini Learning Lesson On The Brain

I've learned a lot about the brain over the past years and one thing I liked was the way information can be easily understood on some web sites I have found. I've used some good information from the Whorsley School and also added my own comments to it, to liven the topic up and have some fun! Here is the link if you are interested: http://www.worsleyschool.net/science/files/brain/page.html

Your brain is pinkish-grey on the outside, and covered in peanut shaped folds and all the other bits of slim, blood, goo and things that are better described by a doctor. Inside, it is a very light shade of yellow. Our brains are very soft, so it needs to be protected by tissues and liquid that surround it, and the bony skull.

The brain has three main parts. The largest is the cerebrum, at the top. The convoluted surface of the cerebrum is called the cerebral cortex, which is only about a third of a centimeter thick, but this is the part that does the thinking and understanding. In some of our cases the old cerebral cortex has let us down, but hey it is thin and small right :) It enables us to learn, remember, and reason. Our cerebrum is actually divided into two halves, called the right and left hemispheres. That's where the phrase developed about using the left side of your brain, or the right side. Each half of the cerebrum is responsible for different tasks. Information is shared between the halves by way of the corpus callosum.

Let's look at what's in a brain, and what each part of the brain does.

CEREBELLUM: It automatically coordinates all of your limb and muscle movements, to help you sit, walk and balance. It's really amazing to think how much brain development a baby goes through as it grows into a child and then adult.

OCCIPITAL LOBE: This part of the brain processes what your eyes see, and turns it into a picture of the world around you. Look out your window right now, that's what is working to allow you to absorb what you see.

PARIETAL LOBE: It controls the sense of touch, and how you use your hands to do things. Hot, cold, smooth and soft are all part of this.

CEREBRUM: This is the top of the brain, covered by the cerebral cortex, which contains your memories and language, and correlates information received from your senses. It controls voluntary movement, emotions, and does the thinking. Yes, it makes a lot of sense to wear your helmet during sports like biking to protect the head.

FRONTAL LOBE: This part of the brain controls your ability to speak. No, people who don't stop talking do not have an over developed frontal lobe!!

TEMPORAL LOBE: This is where signals from our ears are processed, so we can hear. Most of us don't think about the brain when we think about hearing, further support for ear protection.

PONS: Breathing, the regular beating of the heart, and other involuntary activities of the body (the ones that happen without you having to think about it) are controlled here. Yes, this includes snoring!!

BRAIN STEM: This collects all the body-controlling messages from the brain, and passes them on to the rest of the body. Really amazing stuff isn't it!! Kind of like a PC processor.

Let's consider a brain which has been split in half vertically, so we can visualize more structures:

THALAMUS: The thalamus relays incoming messages from your senses to the proper areas of the brain that need to process them.

HYPOTHALAMUS and PITUITARY GLAND: Together these help regulate sexual urges, body temperature, growth, thirst and hunger, maternal behavior (including milk production in mammals), aggression, pleasure, and your 'biological clock', which lets you know when you need to sleep or wake up.

CORPUS CALLOSUM: This portion of the brain is the connection between the two halves of the brain (sometimes called the right and left hemispheres).

The process that your brain uses to store and retrieve information is not well understood, but it works because of the way individual brain cells, called neurons, are connected to each other. Each neuron is covered with dendrites, which are long channels that can receive electrical signals from other neurons. Every neuron makes a connection with the denrites of neurons all around it, using an axon, a fiber for passing signals. In this way, neurons can share information with each other. Every neuron is connected to thousands of others.

The information is actually passed from each axon to a dendrite across a gap called a synapse. The electrical signals trigger neurotransmitters, which are chemicals that move across the gap and stimulate the dendrite, conveying a message from one neuron to another. Every time your brain does something ... think, feel sad, send a signal to move your arm or take a breath ... millions of neurons are sending messages to and from one another. The messages consist of electrical impulses sent down the axons, and chemical messages moving across the synapses.

Neurons have different shapes, depending on the job they do. But *all* neurons share the capability of linking with others in order to pass electrical and chemical messages. As you learn things ... like how to throw a baseball, or how to interpret a poem... your neurons grow more dendrites to become attached to other neurons. The more you repeat that learning, or practice what you've learned, the *stronger* these connections between neurons become. There are over 100,000,000,000,000 possible connections between neurons in the brain, which makes the human brain more powerful than any computer ever made.

If you or someone you know is challenged by ADD, consider the possibilities that exist within the power of the brain, or the brains capability. I have experienced first hand that food, exercise and stimulating my brain by doing things differently all impact and alter my brains capacity for the better.

A Helpful Tip: Knowing what your brain does and how this relates to ADD/ADHD is important. This understanding will allow you to learn more about you and achieve success. Having ADHD and not understanding the neurobiology of ADHD is like having diabetes and not understanding how your blood sugar works.

Chapter 10. My Behavior Changes.

What have I gained? The fruits of success!
Well, to try and explain this could be a project far too large to take on. The ways in which my life has changed could probably not be accurately detailed on paper. I think it is impossible to put to paper, a deep emotional feeling that can only be experienced by myself, regarding my personal experiences. One homework exercise I started doing with Dr. Holly Prochnau was a way of measuring my progression. The below excerpt from my home work exercise is very revealing:

What have I gained?

-   Life experience: this has indeed become a life altering experience. I can look back at this phase of my life and realize that it was one of the key turning points in my life experience.

-   Knowledge of self: I had awakened in my understanding of self. In this process, I had learned and understood what my weaknesses and strengths were as a person. More importantly. I accepted them, which is so important in improving as a person.

-   New people skills (internal & external): The skills I have gained will forever impact my life moving forward. I have become more aware and alert of my thought process when I speak or interact with people now. The skills I have learned allow me to interact with people and build relationships beyond what I was ever capable of previously.

- Happiness: I am a happy man. I have a career, my health, two wonderful children and a great circle of friends and family. I am excited about what the future holds for me.

- A new and improved me: I feel like an improved version of myself. There exists in me, a feeling that I did not get rid of the old me, but instead made some dramatic improvements.

- A more empathetic and sympathetic outlook: the ability to truly understand and feel what empathy and sympathy is, is so powerful. I wonder how I ever managed without this capability previously?

- The ability to be a better father, boyfriend and husband in the future: I am grounded, I understand myself including my strengths, weaknesses and feel very capable and confident. This impacts who I am as a person.

What have I resolved?

- Movement away from a bad marriage: While at the time of my marriage ending I did not realize it. I was in a marriage with the wrong person for the wrong reasons. I never should have gotten married to my now former wife. Today, I see what it is I want and need in a relationship and can avoid the wrong relationship.

- Reduced my anger and deal with it more maturely now: My reaction to situations is now normal, the way it should be. That's not to say I don't and won't get angry, however reacting in a proper way when anger is a more positive and healthier way of living.

- Movement away from narcissistic behavior: I can look back and laugh at some of the things I used to do or say. There is a difference between narcissism and confidence, and thankfully I now realize that.

- Movement away from poor money management: So many people and marriages are impacted by poor money management, myself included. Today, I feel like I have reinvented the fine tuned budget and more importantly, I don't buy on impulse or emotion.

What have I improved?

- Listening skills: I think this is the most improved skill that I have attained. Being able to better listen on a completely different level has really opened up doors for me both personally and in business.

- Understanding of myself: Truly understanding your emotions, thoughts and feeling is so important. You must develop a true understanding and acceptance of your strengths and weaknesses to understand yourself.

What am I aware of?

- I have ADD and need to continue to learn and deal with it. This is not over and never will be. While the major challenge in dealing with ADD is behind me, there will always be work to do. I always need to be aware of this and never lose sight of this focus.

- Others do have a different perception of me and don't share my opinions of self. I have learned that there are a lot of different ways of doing things, feeling and reacting. I don't think there is one right way to do anything, only ways that best suit the situation.

- That I have to manage my anger. Anger is part of everyone's life, how you react to it is what differentiates us. Fortunately, life skills development has allowed me to face this challenge head-on and develop a better way of reacting.

- That I have to consider others with more sympathy and empathy. The ability to do so, has impacted how I converse and the reactions I receive.

In my counseling with Dr. Prochnau, we looked at Brown's Model of ADD. Here are some of the notes I took as I charted my progress:

Noticeable Differences – Taking Concerta Medication & Counseling in relation to Brown's ADD Model

When starting the ADD medication Concerta and counseling, I noticed dramatic differences in relation to Brown's Model of defining and monitoring ADD.

1. Organization, Prioritization & Activating to Work
   - I feel my ability to organize and prioritize was fairly strong prior to taking ADD meds and undergoing counseling.
   - I also feel that initiating work based on organizing and prioritizing was also a strong point.

   - After starting ADD meds and counseling, I now notice a difference in how I maintain organization and priorities when stress or events change and force me to alter my plans or priorities. As an example, I had my kids schedule all planned out in detail. My daughter took ill and required hospitalization. With my Nanny on vacation, this created total chaos personally and with work. I was able to reprioritize quickly, stay focused and avoid letting the situation frustrate me.

2. Focusing, Sustaining Focus, & Shifting Focus To Tasks
   - This was definitely a challenge for me prior to starting ADD meds, coaching and counseling

   - After starting ADD meds, coaching and counseling, the difference was noticeable (meds in less than 48 hours).

   - It may be hard to understand from someone else's position, but it is like I woke up and my senses became alive. I have focus like I have never experienced before in my life. This is an amazing feeling and experience. As an example, I mentioned when my daughter took ill and required hospitalization. This situation impacted work schedules, the kid's schedules/visitation, personal plans and was another stressful event in addition to the separation and divorce proceedings I was experiencing. This would not have been possible previously for me.

3. Regulating Alertness, Sustaining Effort & Processing Speed

- Previous to starting ADD meds, coaching and counseling, I was aware that my alertness and sustaining effort was moderate. However my processing speed was definitely weak.

- After starting ADD meds, coaching and counseling, the difference was noticeable (meds in less than 48 hours).

- I became more alert and was able to sustain that. However, the big difference was processing speed.

- I have become capable of processing at a completely different level, which I was unable to do before. I can now process a person's comment, understand, empathize and sympathize. As an example, previous to staring ADD meds, coaching and counseling I would have to force the thought process of trying to empathize by questioning myself internally. Now, it just happens.

- Another example of better processing was during my daughter's hospitalization. The doctors and nurses would make comments about her condition throughout the day and night. I was able to process these comments, relate them back to previous comments and tie all events and comments together. My processing ability allowed me a clearer understanding of the situation, risks and desired results.

4. Managing Frustration & Modulating Emotions

   - Prior to starting ADD meds, coaching and counseling, managing my emotions was sometimes a challenge

   - After starting ADD meds, coaching and counseling, the difference was noticeable (meds in less than 48 hours).

   - My ability to manage emotions is dramatically different. An example of this would be how I sometimes reacted previously in a situation that frustrated me by slamming a door, throwing something or swearing out loud angrily. I was now able to remain calm and in control and did not over react. I was able to react maturely and accordingly in this situation, and it felt wonderful! I still have to put money into the swear jar in the kitchen on occasion!

5. Monitoring & Self Regulating Action

- Prior to starting ADD meds, coaching and counseling, I did have an issue regarding monitoring and self regulating.

- I believe this was primarily due to having a false sense of self due to ADD

- After starting ADD meds, coaching and counseling, the difference was noticeable in less than 48 hours. The major difference seems to be in having a faster thought process. Such a small amount of time or that fraction of a second of extra time I now had to process made a big difference.

I became much more aware of who I was, the challenges I faced with ADD and my need to maintain my awareness of these challenges to beat them. As an example, whenever a comment or gesture is made by another person, I simply react with all the above noted points in mind. It was like a self regulating software program had been installed in me and it just happened. Of course, I needed to dedicate myself to learning and improving to get to this stage. I am able to regulate, and am fully aware of it. This holds true in emotional situations, how I answer questions or start conversations.

A Helpful Tip: To understand your behavior changes, you must first acknowledge and accept what your behavior weaknesses are.

Chapter 11. Empathy & Sympathy

To me, empathy and sympathy are qualities that allow people to walk in someone else's shoes and truly feel for another person. Children who develop these qualities tend to be more tolerant and compassionate, more understanding of others' needs, and more likely to have good social skills and relationships.

The ability for someone with ADD to truly know, understand and feel what empathy and sympathy is, was one of the biggest challenges I faced. Over the years I can recall reading the definition of empathy and sympathy in dictionaries and in theory, understanding it. However, understanding it and feeling it are two very different things. In fact, understanding the definition of empathy and sympathy is the easy part. Feeling it, now that is when you can truly grasp what empathy and sympathy mean.

I recall many experiences, places and times when I thought that I knew what empathy and sympathy were. I saw someone who drove differently than I did, so I thought they were an idiot or couldn't drive. I listened to my parents drive and meander through getting from point A-to-B with the navigation system in their vehicle wondering how they ever managed without it. I experienced people in business that did things so differently from me, that I couldn't believe they kept their job. In many of these circumstances, my ability to truly feel empathy and sympathy prevented me from understanding a situation and opening my mind to alternate ways of thinking, perceiving, and reacting.

The inability to understand and feel empathy and sympathy was the single biggest challenge for me in my winning my battle against ADD.

The impact of working through the challenge of ADD for me, related heavily to my children. When my marriage came to an end, I was in the process of staring my life over. In this process, I was challenged to work through the many difficulties I was facing. My inability to feel empathy and sympathy impacted my parenting. I was fortunate enough to know and realize this. My parenting was the second most important thing I felt I needed to work on, after self.

A good example of how my lacking the feelings of empathy and sympathy impacted my parenting could be displayed in the simplest of terms. As an example, if my daughter tripped while she was running and ended up with a scrape on her knee, a typical response from me would be, "you'll be OK, you are a big girl now". In reality, all my little girl needed was a hug and the love of her father. In theory, I knew that the scrape she had just suffered on her knee hurt, but I did not understand the feelings she was experiencing. Despite having injured myself playing as a child and an adult more times than I could recollect, her pain meant nothing to me. That all changed after I started Concerta. My ability to actually feel and truly experience empathy and sympathy kicked in, big time! The efforts of counseling and coaching were also a factor in this personal growth. Today when my son scrapes his knee or my daughter drops that toy on her toe, I can feel the emotion they display. What I feel has allowed me to experience a deeper love with my children that I never knew existed.

This ability to empathize and sympathize has also affected relationships with family and friends as well. I referred earlier to listening to my parents drive and meander through getting from point A-to-B using their vehicle navigation system in their vehicle. My Dad was behind the wheel and my Step-Mother was the co-pilot with the map. This was like a front row seat to a live comedy of frustration, or so I thought. As my ability to understand and feel empathy and sympathy grew, my outlook on this situation and many others began to change. As I sat in the back seat listening to my parents and their driving direction discussion, I felt so much and thought about so much. The thoughts that went through my mind we simple, they were complex and they were thought provoking. I finally came to a conclusion after a drive with my parents one day, they managed to get from point A-to-B without my help. In fact they managed to do it every day. Furthermore, they did it in a way that I would never have done. In fact, there was nothing wrong with how they accomplished this. It made me start to think that maybe there was a problem with how I would have driven the same route.

A funny thing happened that day, I learned that there is more than one way to crack an egg, or in this case get from one place to another. I learned what thinking outside the box really meant. The most important experience I went through that day as I sat back and smiled while my parents had an in depth discussion about which highway to take and the ramifications of the alternate route, was that I realized how happy they were, and how good they were for each other. Here I was being critical of people in general, quietly thinking about how foolish they were and during this entire time, I never realized what they were about or what they were experiencing. Previously, I could never have understood this scene. I'm very fortunate today, to be capable of this now, and it has allowed me to re-approach my friendships and family in a more positive and healthy way.

I started experiencing things differently. The use, understanding and feelings of empathy, sympathy and listening skills leads to good relationships, emotional intimacy, and happy marriages. The use may also lead to a conversation partner feeling like she or he is receiving a psychological hug.

I came across some great information on empathy and sympathy online and want to share it at http://changingminds.org/explanations/emotions/empathy.htm

Check this out, very good stuff:

Empathy connects people together. When you empathize with me, my sense of identity is connected to yours. As a result, I feel greater in some way and less alone. I may also start to empathize more with you.

In a therapeutic situation, having someone else really understand how you feel can be a relief, as people with emotional problems often feel very much alone in their different nature. The non-judgmental quality can also be very welcome.

Empathy heals. Therapeutically, it can be a very healing experience for someone to empathize with you. When someone effectively says "I care for you", it also says "I can do that, I can care for myself".

Empathy builds trust. Yet, can also be surprising and confusing. When unexpected, it can initially cause suspicion, but when sustained it is difficult not to appreciate the concern.

Empathy closes the loop. Consider what would happen if you had no idea what the other person felt about what you had said to them. You might say something they hated and you continued as if they understood and agreed.

The more you can empathize, the more you can get immediate feedback on what people are experiencing from your communications with them. As a consequence, you can change what you are saying and doing to get them to feel what you want them to feel.

So how do you do it? How do you find out what other people are feeling? All you have to go on is what they say, how they say it and what they do. If you want to move someone, detecting their emotional state is the first step. If you can feel that state, then that detection is even more accurate. When you can sense their emotion, you can then use this to move them in the direction you want them to take. I say this with the assumption that moving someone in a direction is done with good intent. Otherwise, it will likely backfire on you.

The trick in spotting feelings is to pay close attention to changes in the other person in response to external events. If you say "How are you?" and the corners of their mouth turn down and their voice tone goes flat, then you might detect, all is not well.

The better you are at spotting small changes, the greater your potential ability at empathizing. Watch for small changes on the face. Watch for lower-body movements when the upper-body is under conscious control. Listen for tension in the voice and an emphasis on specific words. Listen for emotional words.

To avoid getting swamped by their emotions, learn to dip in and out of the association that makes you feel what they do. Go in, test the temperature and then get out to a place where you can think more rationally. Unless you are really sure, it can be a good idea to reflect back to the other person what you are sensing of their feelings, to check that you have got it right. After all, the only person who can confirm empathy is the person whose emotions are being sensed.

Reflecting back has an effect, typically leading the other person to appreciate that you really care about them and thus, increasing their trust in you. Empathy is far more effective when it is offered, as opposed to being sought.

Just to reiterate the obvious, the usual caveat applies here; taking advantage of someone who is upset breaks many social rules and negative manipulation is likely to lead to trouble.

A Helpful Tip: To truly empathize and sympathize at a deep level, will allow you to develop and maintain rewarding and life long relationships in all areas of your life

Chapter 12. The Work Doesn't Stop

If anyone stops growing or learning, that person is in big trouble! Whether you have ADD or not, one needs to continue to evolve and become a better person. As my ADD coach told me, "the work doesn't stop". I continue to work on me and think of this not only as a process that allows me to win the challenge against ADD, but also because I want to continually work at being better person. I'm happy with me, however I want to challenge myself and reap the rewards of life. In turn, I feel that will create better relationships with my children, family and friends. In continuing to work on me, I determined there were many things that I could do to grow and evolve. These include:

Setting Goals

The process of goal setting and targets allows me to choose where I want to go in my life, because it is my life after all. By knowing what I want to achieve, I know what I have to focus on and what it will take to do it.

Goal setting is now used everywhere by people in sports, the most successful business people we see in the papers and online and by winners in all fields no matter where we look. Goal setting allows us to create a long term road map and come up with the baby steps we need to make in order to get there. By goal setting, it enables us to concentrate on the task at hand, stay focused and succeed. By setting our goals, we can evaluate our progress and feel that achievement when we complete the goal.

Setting goals can also impact self confidence. It's a great feeling when we achieving goals we set out to accomplish. It makes us want to do more, because we believe in ourselves. It sure impacts me positively!

We can set goals for so many different things. The most obvious goal is to first decide what it is we want to accomplish? The next step is to break down the steps it will take to achieve that goal, into baby steps or small steps. This helps to create that road map to success and will give us the plan we need to follow to win. Try to set goals in as many areas of your life as possible.

I use something my ADD coach Pete Quily supplied me, it's called The Wheel of Life. Remember that olds song:

"The wheels of life are turning so much faster, the restless hands of time pass me by"

Yes, these are the lyrics to the classic 70's hit "The Wheels of Life" by Gino Vanelli.

The wheels of life can entail many things and have different meaning to people. To me, the wheel of life is a great tool that benefits people with and without ADD. The wheel of life is about balancing the different and key things that are a part of your life. I use the categories in this tool to evaluate my life and set goals. The 8 categories of analysis are, in no particular order;

1) Career
2) Money

3) Health
4) Friends & Family
5) Significant Other
6) Personal Growth
7) Fun & Recreation
8) Physical Environment.

It is about analyzing each of these categories in your life to determine if your life is balanced. Draw a circle and divide it into 8 equal pieces of pie. Each piece of pie in the circle represents one of the above 8 categories. Color in each category, the further you color towards the edge of the circle, the more pleased you are with this life category. Once you have colored each of the 8 life categories, you will have a new edge of the circle. This edge could be smooth all the way around, but will likely have some rough edges because you are human after all. If any of the categories are not balanced, the wheel won't roll too smoothly, so to speak. It's up to you to smoothen out that wheel rotation and work on the parts of your life that need improvement.

We all need to improve continually. Understanding who you are, what your strengths consist of and what challenges you is an important part of this process.

When I set goals within these categories, I create the baby steps required to build up to achieving my goals. This includes reprioritizing sometimes. This will also ensure help you to reconfirm your goals and make sure this is what you are truly interested in achieving. This is YOUR life!

During the time when I am focused on my goals, I also do a self review every Sunday, kind of like a self tune-up. I have a piece of paper with the below criteria on it. I'll take a few minutes to read through it and ask myself the questions on it, and answer them honestly. Basically, a self grading system. Here is the list that I use:

- Avoiding Conflict – did I avoid conflict in certain situations? What could I have done better? What did I do well this week and what was the result?

- Fun – whatever I did, did I have fun? If not, why?

- Problems – what problems did I encounter and how did these occur? How can they be avoided?

- Value – What value did I offer in particular situations, actions or conversations?

- Win-Win – What situations was I involved in where my efforts could have been better and benefited all?

- Patience – Did I lack patience in a particular experience? Where did I show patience successfully?

- Intimacy – Did I allow myself to communicate and open up in intimate situations, letting someone else get what they needed from me?

- Defensiveness – was I defensive or over reactive in any situations? If yes, why could this have happened?

- Dealing with Change – What changed? Why did it change? How did I handle or manage this change?

- Familiarity – Is my familiarity crossing the line of complacency? Is it OK or do I need to shake it up?

- Balance – is my life balanced? If not, what needs to change in my life the achieve balance?

- Kindness – did I perform any acts of kindness? If not, could I have been kinder in a situation?

- Celebration – did I take any time to celebrate what I have in my life and appreciate my surroundings?

- Laughter – was I laughing? If not, why not?!

- Disorganization – how was my organization and structure recently?

- Telling myself the Truth – was I kidding myself and not being honest with a decision I had to make?

- Hard times – how did I react? Good? Bad?

- Thoughtfulness – what thoughtful actions or comments did I experience? Was it me? Was it someone else who commented toward me?

- Rewarding Yourselves – what is my reward for doing something well? We all deserve a reward.

- Being Spontaneous – did I loosen up and just roll with it, live on the edge a little?

It only takes 10 minutes to sit and think through this list. However, that 10 minutes is a valuable educational thinking process that helps to determine my direction and actions for the coming week. It makes me aware and alert of all the criteria by which I measure myself.

A Helpful Tip: Revisit your progress regularly. The work will never stop and by not using a Checklist to make sure you are on track, you could run the risk of becoming complacent and falling back into old habits.

Chapter 13. Time Management

Of the many potential challenges a person can face with ADD, I have been lucky enough not to have been burdened by time management. Within the functionality of time management, there have always been some challenges, like prioritizing. Fortunately I learned about time management at a very young age and these lessons have always remained with me. Ironically, we really can't manage time, we can only manage our selves in time periods.

Every day, I see friends, Moms, Dads and people working who believe they are not wasting any time and that they have time management under control. "I'm very organized" is what I hear an awful lot of. Yet for most people, their days end up being scattered, too busy and often unproductive. We all end up running around like chickens with their heads cut off, as the saying goes.

That can be very frustrating, I've been there. The idea of time management has been around for ages, I'm sure it was used in some form hundreds of years ago, some how.

Once we all realize time can't be managed and that time is actually out of our control, we can focus on managing ourselves as best as we can within time. Ah, suddenly time already feels a little more in control when I say that and understand it.

I've heard it before and remember reading it a few times in various places, "time management is actually self management". Within time management or self management we need to be able to set goals, plan, delegate, organize, direct and control.

There are a lot of tools and strategies we can use to manage our time, gain control of our lives stop the cycle of wasting time and getting stressed out. Through the coaching process, Pete Quily offered me the opportunity to do a presentation to an ADD support group that Pete chaired and managed. I was nervous about this at first, but after giving it some thought I started to feel that this was a great opportunity. It would force me to revisit the principles of my own time management, it would likely result in the refinement of that process and it just may offer some assistance to someone else in the support group. I came across some great information online to help me build a template to speak to, like much of the below detail from The University of Nebraska http://www.ianrpubs.unl.edu/epublic/pages/publicat ionD.jsp?publicationId=860

Here is an outline of what I presented to the group.

Time Management Tips

SPEND TIME PLANNING AND ORGANIZING. Using time to think and plan is time well-spent. In fact, if you fail to take time to plan, you are in effect, planning to fail. Organize in a way that makes sense to you. If you need color and pictures, use a lot on your calendar or planning book. Some people need to have papers filed away; others get their creative energy from their piles. So forget the "shoulds" and organize your way.

SET GOALS. Goals give your life, and the way you spend your time, direction. When asked the secret to amassing such a fortune, one of the famous Hunt brothers from Texas replied: "First you've got to decide what you want." Set goals which are specific, measurable, realistic and achievable. Your optimum goals are those which cause you to "stretch" but not "break" as you strive for achievement. Goals can give creative people a much-needed sense of direction.

PRIORITIZE. Use the 80-20 Rule, 80 percent of the reward comes from 20 percent of the effort. The trick to prioritizing is to isolate and identify that valuable 20 percent. Once identified, prioritize time to concentrate your work on those items with the greatest reward. Prioritize by color, number or letter, whichever method makes the most sense to you. Flagging items with a deadline is another idea for helping you stick to your priorities.

USE A TO DO LIST. Some people thrive using a daily "To Do" list in which they list either the last "To Do" from the previous day or first thing in the morning. Such people may combine a To Do list with a calendar or schedule. Others prefer a "running" To Do list which is continuously being updated. Or, you may prefer a combination of the two previously described To Do lists. Whatever method works is best for you. Don't be afraid to try a new system — you just might find one that works even better than your present one!

BE FLEXIBLE. Allow time for interruptions and distractions. Time management experts often suggest planning for just 50 percent or less of one's time. With only 50 percent of your time planned, you will have the flexibility to handle interruptions and the unplanned "emergency." When you expect to be interrupted, schedule routine tasks. Save (or make) larger blocks of time for your priorities. When interrupted, reprioritize by asking, "What is the most important thing I can be doing with my time right now?" to help you get back on track.

CONSIDER YOUR BIOLOGICAL PRIME TIME. That's the time of day when you are at your best. Are you a morning person, a night owl, or a late afternoon whiz? Knowing your best time and planning to use that time of day for your priorities (if possible) is effective time management.

DO THE RIGHT THING RIGHT. Noted management expert, Peter Drucker, says "doing the right thing is more important than doing things right." Doing the right thing is effectiveness; doing things right is efficiency. Focus first on effectiveness (identifying what is the right thing to do), then concentrate on efficiency (doing it right).

ELIMINATE THE URGENT. Urgent tasks have short-term consequences while important tasks are those with long-term, goal-related implications. Work towards reducing the urgent things you must do so you'll have time for your important priorities. Flagging or highlighting items on your To Do list or attaching a deadline to each item may help keep important items from becoming urgent emergencies.

PRACTICE THE ART OF INTELLIGENT NEGLECT. Eliminate from your life trivial tasks or those tasks which do not have long-term consequences for you. Can you delegate or eliminate any of your To Do list? Work on those tasks which you alone can do.

AVOID BEING A PERFECTIONIST. Who in the world can be considered capable of producing anything perfect? Yes, some things need to be closer to perfect than others, but perfectionism, paying unnecessary attention to detail, can be a form of procrastination.

CONQUER PROCRASTINATION. When you are avoiding something, break it into smaller tasks and do just one of the smaller tasks or set a timer and work on the big task for just 15 minutes. By doing a little at a time, eventually you'll reach a point where you'll want to finish. Before you realize it, you will be finished.

LEARN TO SAY "NO." For some, it is so hard to say no. Focusing on your goals may help. Blocking time for important, but often not scheduled priorities such as family and friends can also help. But first you must be convinced that you and your priorities are important — that seems to be the hardest part in learning to say no. Once convinced of their importance, saying no to the unimportant in life gets easier.

REWARD YOURSELF. Even for small successes, celebrate achievement of goals. Promise yourself a reward for completing each task, or finishing the total job. Then keep your promise to yourself and indulge in your reward. Doing so will help you maintain the necessary balance in life between work and play. As Ann McGee-Cooper says, "If we learn to balance excellence in work with excellence in play, fun, and relaxation, our lives become happier, healthier, and a great deal more creative."

A Helpful Tip: Try an experiment, write down a list of five things you need to do this week. Prioritize them and schedule them throughout the week. Once you have completed "to do" tasks, reflect back and ask yourself if using time management and organization helped you?

Chapter 14. Kids......A New Perspective

A person with ADD who is raising kids can be challenged, yet this challenge can be met and overcome. In an odd way, being diagnosed with ADD made me a better father. It forced me to be much more aware, alert and the personal growth that I have experienced has benefited my parenting.

I am a single Dad, with equal custody of my son and daughter. Single parents and their children continue to become a rapidly increasing part of the population in North America. Much of the initial research on single parent families focused on single mothers due to the father's absence. More recently, single fathers with equal custody are starting to become a normal thing. Today's family units provide a alternative to the traditional nuclear families, which seem to be going the way of dinosaurs. The traditional nuclear family is now the minority in North America.

Single fathers have found ways to work, supervise children, clean the house and do the laundry. They are able to perform homemaking tasks such as cooking, cleaning, and shopping outside what we are accustomed to. In fact, homemaking is a major part of single father's roles. Fathers today are more familiar with these roles in home, which is a big change from generations of the past. I'd say that's a good thing, as would most women.

Ten years ago, if I would have stopped at a Physic's for a palm reading to peer into my future, I would have laughed if I was told I would be part of the single parent demographic and have to deal with

ADD. Well, this is my reality and it really is unbelievable the many roads one can take to achieve happiness. The major factor in my happiness is definitely my two incredible children.

I am aware of the challenges I face with ADD, as I am of my weaknesses. What I needed to do was give a lot of thought to how I was parenting and how I would influence and teach my children. More importantly, what would my children see and learn by simply watching me or emulating my actions.

What a powerful experience! As if it weren't already a big enough responsibility to bring up children, I was now facing parenthood wondering about every little thing I did or said and how it would impact my kids as a result of having ADD. In retrospect, I believe that I over thought this when pondering how I was going to move forward. However, at least I didn't under think it.

How was I going to approach this challenge? Well, I figured the best approach involved three steps:

1. Understand my challenges with ADD – I literally got a pen and a piece of paper and wrote them down

2. Understand how my challenges could impact my children negatively – I was worried at first, but that concern turned into my motivation to ensure I would be the best father I could.

3. Work on dealing with my challenges of ADD – I needed to improve, learn and see real results in how I parented.

It was time to put the plan into action! As I have mentioned previously, I believed that I was a good father but I needed to become a better father. The symptoms that I was most challenged by were:

Activating to Work – getting myself to perform that action was always a challenge, primarily with reprioritization.

Focusing and Sustaining Focus – easily I would lose track of what I was involved with, including a conversation, work task or listening.

Processing Speed – I just seemed to be a thought behind everyone else or a little too slow in coming up with a response.

Managing Frustration & Emotions – I was easily frustrated with tasks, actions of others and had a temper.

Narcissism – I has a false sense of who I was and my capabilities.

With my challenges identified, I had to now fully understand how these could impact my children negatively. I once again picked up pen and paper and started the list of my concerns which included:

a) What would my children see when they looked at me or observed?

b) What habits would they pick up that they had learned from me?

c) How did I want my children to react emotionally?

d) What kind of temperament should a child display?

e) How could I react when their emotions or temperament needed correcting?

f) What kind of focus and concentration habits would they develop?

g) What would their thought process be?

h) How could I teach them to think?

i) What could I do to teach them about humility yet build confidence and positive attitudes?

j) How could I establish the basics of organization and build upon that?

So many questions and thoughts were running through my mind. After I gave this a tremendous amount of thought, I realized that the challenges I was facing with ADD and working on already were the same as parenting with ADD. I was already working on the challenges with my ADD coach, reading books and doing a ton of research on line. It was then that I realized I was on track and heading in the right direction. Like realizing that I was also being too hard on myself when I came off my medication, I was also too hard on myself regarding parenting. I would have rather been too hard on myself then not hard enough.

One of the great experiences in parenting are the little things that your kids surprise you with. It could be an "I love you" or a hug, or an action that just makes your day when you least expect it. As I started to deal with ADD and win my battle, parenting also became easier. I found that success for me as a parent was based on two items, planning and review.

Planning is very important when it comes to any one's life. With ADD it is even more important. Time can go by quickly and without planning activities with my children, I found that days and weeks would go by, until I realized that I needed to plan more regarding play time, education, talking, down time and the many aspects of parenting that must occur. While many things will happen naturally within the everyday activities of a busy life, I found I needed to take time and schedule more. As my son started to learn to read, I dedicated fifteen minutes a day three times per week to assisting him. Three things happened. Firstly, my sons reading skills improved. Second, my son was obviously thrilled with the time we spent together and that enhanced the relationship. Third, I had a great time doing it!

Taking the time to plan and schedule activities with other kids for playtime, reading, outdoor activities, movies and many other things were and are an important goal for me as a parent to achieve.

As an adult with ADD, I'm now very aware of signs and signals that my children could have ADD as well. I've really looked into how to recognize ADD in kids and what to do if required in the future. I found that CHADD (Children and Adults With Attention-Deficit/Hyperactivity Disorder) http://www.chadd.org/ is an excellent web site for general information and gaining knowledge. I found it to be very important in my personal growth to understand my children and be sure if the situation did arise in the future regarding ADD, that I would be able to understand a diagnosis process, medications and alternately, misdiagnosis and medicating when not required.

This is information is taken directly from the CHADD web site:

"When A Child Has ADD, What Can a Parent Do To Help?

Often, when a child is diagnosed with AD/HD, the first response from his or her concerned parent is, "What can I do about it?" Although life with your child may at times seem challenging, it is important to remember that children with ADD/ADHD can and do succeed. As a parent, you can help create home and school environments that improve your child's chances for success. The earlier you address your child's problems, the more likely you will be able to prevent school and social failure and associated problems such as underachievement and poor self-esteem that may lead to delinquency or drug and alcohol abuse.

Early intervention holds the key to positive outcomes for your child. Here are some ways to get started:

Learn all you can about AD/HD. There is a great deal of information available on the diagnosis and treatment of AD/HD. It is up to you to act as a good consumer and *learn* to distinguish the "accurate" information from the "inaccurate." But how can you sort out what will be useful and what will not? In general, it is good to be wary about ads claiming to cure AD/HD.

Make sure your child has a comprehensive assessment. To complete the diagnostic process, make sure your child has a comprehensive assessment that includes medical, educational, and psychological evaluations and that other disorders that either mimic or commonly occur with AD/HD have been considered and ruled out.

Become an effective case manager. Keep a record of all information about your child. This includes copies of all evaluations and documents from any meetings concerning your child. You might also include information about AD/HD, a record of your child's prior treatments and placements, and contact information for the professionals who have worked with your child.

Take an active role in forming a team that understands AD/HD and wants to help your child. Meetings at your child's school should be attended by the principal's designee, as well as a special educator and a classroom teacher that knows your child. You, however, have the right to request input at these meetings from others that understand AD/HD or your child's special needs. These include your child's physician, the school psychologist, and the nurse or guidance counselor from your child's school. If you have consulted other professionals, such as a psychiatrist, educational advocate or behavior management specialist, the useful information they have provided should also be made available at these meetings. A thorough understanding of your child's strengths and weaknesses and how AD/HD affects him will help you and members of this team go on to develop an appropriate and effective program that takes into account his or her AD/HD.

Learn all you can about AD/HD and your child's educational rights. The more knowledge you have about your child's rights under education laws - the Individuals with Disabilities Education Act (IDEA in USA) and Section 504 of the Rehabilitation Act (USA)- the better the chance that you will maximize his or her success. Each state has a parent training and information center that can help you learn more about your child's rights. (visit www.taalliance.org/centers to find the center in your state). Similar resources are also available in Canada.

Become your child's best advocate. You may have to represent or protect your child's best interest in school situations, both academic and behavioral. Become an active part of the team that determines what services and placements your child receives.

How to Make Life at Home Easier

Join a support group. Parents will find additional information, as well as support, by attending local CHADD meetings where available. You can find the nearest chapter to your home on http://www.chadd.org chapter locator.

Seek professional help. Ask for help from professionals, particularly if you are feeling depressed, frustrated and exhausted. Helping yourself feel less stressed will benefit your child as well.

Work together to support your child. It is important that all of the adults that care for your child (parents, grandparents, relatives, and babysitters) agree on how to approach or handle your child's problem behaviors. Working with a professional, if needed, can help you better understand how to work together to support your child.

Learn the tools of successful behavior management. Parent training will teach you strategies to change behaviors and improve your relationship with your child. Identify parent training classes in your community through your local parent information and resource center (http://www.federalresourcecenter.org/frc/TAGuide/welcome.htm) or parent training and information center (http://www.taalliance.org/centers).

Find out if you have AD/HD. Many parents of children with AD/HD often discover that they have AD/HD when their child is diagnosed. Parents with AD/HD may need the same types of evaluation and treatment that they seek for their children in order to function at their best. AD/HD in the parent may make the home more chaotic and affect parenting skills.

Parent training will help you learn to:

Focus on certain behaviors and provide clear, consistent expectations, directions and limits. Children with AD/HD need to know exactly what others expect from them. They do not perform well in ambiguous situations that don't specify exactly what is expected and that require they read between the lines. Working with a professional can help you narrow the focus to a few specific behaviors and help you set limits, and consistently follow through.

Set up an effective discipline system. Parents should learn proactive, not reactive discipline methods that teach and reward appropriate behavior and respond to misbehavior with alternatives such as "time out" or loss of privileges.

Help your child learn from his or her mistakes. At times, negative consequences will arise naturally out of a child's behavior. However, children with AD/HD have difficulty making the connection between their behaviors and these consequences. Parents can help their child with AD/HD make these connections and learn from his or her mistakes.

How to Boost Your Child's Confidence

Tell your child that you love and support him or her unconditionally. There will be days when you may not believe this yourself. Those will be the days when it is even more important that you acknowledge the difficulties your child faces on a daily basis, and express your love. Let your child know that you will get through the smooth and rough times together.

Assist your child with social skills. Children with AD/HD may be rejected by peers because of hyperactive, impulsive or aggressive behaviors. Parent training can help you learn how to assist your child in making friends and learning to work cooperatively with others.

Identify your child's strengths. Many children with AD/HD have strengths in certain areas such as art, athletics, computers or mechanical ability. Build upon these strengths, so that your child will have a sense of pride and accomplishment. Make sure that your child has the opportunity to be successful while pursuing these activities and that his strengths are not undermined by untreated AD/HD. Also, avoid, as much as possible, targeting these activities as contingencies for good behavior or withholding them, as a form of punishment, when your child with AD/HD misbehaves.

Set aside a daily "special time" for your child. Constant negative feedback can erode a child's self-esteem. A "special time," whether it's an outing, playing games, or just time spent in positive interaction, can help fortify your child against assaults to self-worth.

A Helpful Tip: Try planning and scheduling activities well in advance with children. It relieves the pressure to plan spontaneously and the kids become more fulfilled, happy and receive the attention they crave.

Chapter 15. Exercise & Nutrition

The constant message advocating exercise and a balanced diet is a part of our daily lives. We see the weight loss commercial on TV and radio ads for the gym that will have you looking better in 4 weeks and don't forget about the ads for diet pills, power shakes, energy bars and the many other miracle products out there.

On my road of experience with ADD I can look back and identify many points along the way that were milestones, where change took place and a shift for the better occurred within me. One milestone that was a key factor in my personal growth, was physical health. I view exercise and nutrition as the building blocks of both physical and emotional health. Exercise is unique to each individual and with so many different ways to participate, there are a lot of options to consider. For me, I have always been very active in athletics so the process of finding an exercise routine that worked for me was very enjoyable. One thing remains true in almost every person's life no matter who you are, nothing is better than exercise and balanced eating habits. I hate the word diet!

While I exercise in many different ways, the two consistent aspects of my exercise program are running and weight lifting. When I hit the point of where I realized that ADD was messing up my life, I was also approaching a personal weight level that I was disgusted with when I looked in the mirror. In retrospect, I consider my self very fortunate to not have had a serious weight problem. However, the fact remained that I needed to lose 40 pounds and I looked like hell.

My initial running goal was to maintain a reasonable pace for a minimum of 30 minutes. Easy stuff I thought, but it wasn't. I needed to run, take a walking break, run then take another walking break and continued with this for a few weeks. The day did arrive when I was able to continue running and complete my run from start to finish. My first start to finish run was 6km, or just under 4 miles. I started to increase that distance and moved my distance to 7km, then worked my way up to 8km. My next goal was to make it to the 10km distance. I soon achieved that and even started running competitive 10km races. In fact, I achieved a personal best 10km time of 42:26.

When I weight lifted at the gym in the past, I had the ability to build mass and size very easily, naturally. This could be viewed as a blessing by many athletes who intentionally try to build size with weights. However for me, it was a not a blessing. As a result, I needed to re-learn how to weight lift to achieve my goal of strengthening and toning, not building mass. The program I ended up working with was one with light weights and a high repetition program. This helped me to avoid building mass, focus on taking weight off and improve my muscular tone. As an example, instead of doing 3 sets of bicep curls to work my arms by lifting 40 pound dumbbells 8 times each, I now will do 5 sets of curls with 25 pound dumbbells 12 times each.

As I started to work towards my goals, there were many changes that I started to notice in myself. The first and most obvious was I was losing my excess weight, which was also tied to healthy nutrition. The second impact was that I started to become much more energized throughout my workday and weekends. I had more energy to complete my workday and more energy to play with my kids. This energy also translated into a clearer and sharper mind for me, which is very important in the challenge one faces with ADD.

When my mind is clear from exercising, I can focus more, I can think in a more logical and structured fashion and that allows me to attain better results in all areas of my life. In this busy world, there will be times when work, family or unplanned events will draw you away from your required exercise. I have learned two very important lessons regarding this, the first being:

1) Schedule it
2) If I don't do it I will not function at my capacity.

I can not express the importance of scheduling my exercise times and actions. I consider my exercise to be more important an event than a work. If I don't exercise, all the other actions, engagements, meetings or what ever I am doing will suffer. Exercise is the pin that holds my hinge in place. If I don't schedule the exercise activity and time, everything else seems too important or too busy, or so I think. That then leaves me in a place in which I do not function properly. It really makes sense for me and there are many reasons to begin or maintain a regular exercise program.

An improved physical activity level may lower your blood pressure, and also prevent heart attacks and strokes. You should talk to your doctor about this. Numerous medical studies have shown that an exercise improves the quality of life. Regular aerobic exercise, such as walking, jogging or riding a bike has been shown to lower blood pressure and deliver many other benefits as well. Additionally, something as simple as a regular walking program can improve your blood circulation, make your breathing better and will help your body and mind get into in better shape and stay there.

There are so many other activities we can participate in like hiking, a simple exercise video on TV, swimming, aerobics classes at the gym or community center and sports such as tennis, squash, basketball, baseball, ice hockey and so on. If you're about to start on an exercise program, here are some tips on getting started:

- Keep mixing it up and refining it. Our bodies will usually respond and you can push yourself to do more

- Schedule EVERYTHING! It will make your life so much easier and enjoyable.

  Here are some great tips from Take It To Another Level
  http://www.takeittoanotherlevel.com/testing-server/fitness.php

- If you haven't been exercising regularly, check with your doctor before beginning any new program. If you have high blood pressure or other risk factors for heart disease, work with your doctor to determine a safe and effective exercise plan.

- Read up on the sport or activity you've chosen.

- Avoid dehydration by drinking plenty of water before, during and after exercising.

- If it's too hot to exercise outdoors, find an indoor facility or work out early in the morning to avoid the hottest part of the day.

- Wear comfortable shoes and clothing that is appropriate for the activity.

- Begin your exercise regimen slowly and steadily, and have plenty of patience. Don't overdo it. Trying to do too much too fast could lead to muscle strain, back problems, or any other number of joint or muscle disorders.

- If you're getting into weight lifting, allow your muscles the chance to ease into the workout regimen.

- If you're getting into aerobic exercise, observe the workout session to determine if the class is right for you. Consider beginning with low-impact aerobics, rather than the more demanding high-impact aerobics.

- If you're getting into running, warm up to loosen your muscles before a run and stretch only after. Hold the stretch position for 15 to 20 seconds. Avoid a bouncing stretch.

- Find someone experienced in fitting shoes for the activity you've chosen to avoid damage or strain to your feet and legs.

If you're considering investing in exercise equipment, know what your fitness goals are to select the appropriate equipment:

- To improve aerobic fitness, consider a treadmill, a stair climber, a rowing machine or a stationary bike.

- To improve muscular strength, consider a home gym or joining a gym or fitness club.

and before you invest:

- Make sure you have enough space to use the equipment properly. If the equipment must be set up and put away for each exercise session, be sure it does not deter to your fitness program.

- Make sure you are comfortable with the movements and exercise required, including concentration and coordination needed, and learning curve. With a strength training machine, make sure changing weights is exceedingly simple. With a rowing machine, make sure there isn't undue strain on your back. The equipment should fit you.

- Don't overbuy expensive features or gadgets that you won't use frequently.

- Talk with other exercisers and fitness professionals.

- Don't skimp on the basics, such as sturdy construction, and smooth, quiet operation.

- Try out the equipment before making a purchase, and try it more than once to check for stability, structural integrity and ease of operation. For cardio machines, spend at least 20 minutes trying different programs; for strength equipment, do a set of 10 repetitions.

- Try the top-of-the-line equipment, so you can compare the quality of features as you check other brands.

- Shop around, and compare prices, as well as features.

- Investigate various models and manufacturers; and understand the differences in equipment, construction and warranty.

- Check the equipment's warranty, and know what's required for the equipment to be repaired or serviced under warranty. Find out if the warranty is from the manufacturer or from the retailer.

- Find out about assembly and setup, service and maintenance.

- If you are buying online, ensure the company is reputable and will ship the equipment safely so that it isn't damaged in transit.

Good luck as you begin and sustain an important element of healthy living. You'll soon notice a difference in the way you or someone you know with ADD feels, works and eventually succeeds in overcoming the challenges of ADD.

Nutrition has also played an important factor in my progress to date. We have all heard the phrase, "you are what you eat." I believe in this whole heartedly. As an example, if I stop at McDonalds for a Big Mac, pop and fries, that meal selection stays with me and haunts me. It impacts my energy levels, which relates directly to how I will perform that day. Also, I can feel it just sitting in the pit of my stomach. Alternatively, if I choose to stop and eat some vegetables, maybe a lean piece of chicken breast and a glass of milk, the impact on my energy and how that relates to my performance of activity and thinking is dramatically different. It is much better.

The choices I have the ability to make, will and do make a difference. The choices I make relate to my attitude, so refresh your memory by going back to the beginning of Chapter 1 and taking 30 seconds to re-read "Attitude " by Charles Swindell. DO IT!! .... Welcome back, I really find reviewing "Attitude" helps me to focus. I read it almost every day.

A Helpful Tip: Remember the old phrase "you are what you eat". Proper nutrition and exercise need to be seriously considered. Try to plan out your meals and snacks in one week increments. This will eliminate last minute scrambling for meals and avoid quick fast food meals.

Chapter 16. Learn To Relax

Relaxation, sounds very easy. In reality most adults, whether challenged by ADD or not, couldn't relax if they tried. Learning to relax is an important skill more people should learn. I just used the term "learn", because in my case I had no idea how to relax. I had to learn how to turn it off and what to do in order to accomplish this.

My coaching sessions with Pete Quily were very instrumental in learning how to relax. Each week during our coaching time, Pete would challenge me with learning a new way to relax and planning that relaxtion activity regularly throughout the week. Little things like breathing deeply or picturing a quiet peacful place in my minds eye. Seriously, I was the first to cringe my brow and wonder if this was a little too odd? However, I gave it a chance and it was effective. Soon enough I progressed into a relaxation web site that took about 5 minutes. I would click on http://www.positivepause.com/ and watch the on line relaxation video in the middle of the day when work got a little hectic and stressfull.

As time progressed, I soon realized the only effective way to relax, was to set aside time for myself to relax. Relaxation can be many different things for many different people. For me, it could be a nice bottle of red wine, the sunset at the beach, turning on some easy going music and lighting a fire or some candles. There are many different ways a person can relax and each person has their own preference. Another great way to relax that I learned through coaching, was to reward myself. After my coaching sessions, I would have assignments or tasks to work on. Once I achieved my goals, it was important to reward myself. Rewarding myself was not about expensive gifts of self indulgence, but more about a little treat for accomplishing what I set out to do. For me, maybe it was a Smartie Blizzard from Dairy Queen, or treating myself to a nice bottle of wine I had saved for a special occasion. I also rewarded myself with massage, turning off my computer and ending my work day a little earlier on a Friday and treating myself to some jumbo scalops marinated in a ginger-soy-honey marinade.

I recall many times when I was very stressed out from work or life, and I would hit one of my scheduled times to relax during the day. That small 5 minute time period when I chose to relax allowed me to refocus, relieve stress, clear my mind and get my day back on track. The key to relaxation for me was and is based on three factors:

1) Scheduling a specific time to relax daily and

2) Identifying when I need to relax.

3) Doing it.

Too often in the past I would just endure stress and overwhelming challenges. As with many lessons in life, hindsight offers all the answers. Learning to harness and take advantage of my foresight proved to be very valuable.

Understanding that if I didn't relax, I would not be productive or effective made me realize the importance of actually relaxing. Not taking that time to relax resulted in increased stress, burning out and that would inevitably impact my health.

Learn to relax, learn what your "relaxers" are and schedule time for yourself. It will improve the quality of your life and dramatically assist with winning the challenge against ADD. For me, relaxtion resulted in stress management.

Try these ten relaxation tips I found online at Squidoo http://www.squidoo.com/hotgifts

1. Make time to relax! I know, there is so much to do, and if you're not doing it you're thinking about doing it. To relax you need to give yourself permission, to grant yourself a little time in which to practice. But it sure beats a heart attack! It also beats anxiety and exhaustion. Don't waste your life on feeling exhausted. Fifteen minutes a day of relaxation practice can help a lot.

2. Carry a small notebook with you everywhere and leave it next to your bed at night. Even have it with you when you're practicing to relax. Jot down anything that occurs to you that needs to be done. Go through the list now and then. Cross off what you really don't need to do, and you'll feel lighter. Then as you work your way through the list check off what you've done, and you'll feel more in control of your life.

3. Sleep! If you have trouble sleeping, you've already tried various techniques. Here are some that worked for me. Before trying to sleep do something you love to do and don't have time for during the day. Maybe you love to read in bed for at least half

an hour before you sleep, or listen to music or watch sports highlights. I feel like I've given myself a gift in learning to do this, and that feeling is good and relaxing. Keep that notebook next to your bed for jotting down stray emergency thoughts!

Sometimes I place a cold cloth over my eyes to help me drift off. There's something soothing about the cool soft weight. Keep the heat turned down, adjust the light the way you like it, and let go.

4. When you get home from work, take fifteen minutes for yourself. Put the kids somewhere safe; you'll work something out! Lie flat on your back (I prefer the floor). First, bring your knees up so that your lower back touches the floor. Lower your legs straight out and your back will be in a good position for relaxing. Let your feet flop outwards, have your arms a little out from your sides with the palms facing up. Now go through your whole body mentally, focusing your attention on one area at a time. Think "relax" at each area. Start with one foot: the sole of the foot, the top of the foot, the ankle, the front of the calf, the back of the calf, and so on. Then the other leg. Then the abdomen, the buttocks, the lower back. You get the idea. For your arms, start with your fingers and work your way up. Finish with the throat, the back of the neck, the jaw, nostrils, eyelids, temples and forehead.

Someone might have to wake you up, but you'll be very relaxed! And good company for the rest of the evening.

5. Try open-eyed meditation. One way of doing this is by gazing softly (not staring) at a candle flame.

Darken the room, light a candle, sit comfortably and gaze at the flame. The aim is to have a focus for the mind. So when your mind wanders, gently bring your attention back to the flame. Calming the mind is the basis of all relaxation techniques, and that's why you'll feel warm and relaxed after doing the exercise.

6. The home spa! Of course, the real thing is fantastic, but we're talking about everyday life here. Again, it's all about giving yourself permission both to give yourself time, and to give yourself something pleasurable.

First step: set aside the time. Second step: arrange for no interruptions for an hour. Third step: take all the paraphernalia you need, go into the bathroom and close the door. Just for the record, this really works guys. Don't think of this as something for women only, let go and try something new. I suggest putting the music on first. Then arrange your candles and light them. Turn off the light and start the bath running. Add aromatherapy bath salts or bubble bath and breathe deeply. Turn off the water and step into the tub. Lie down. Sigh! Close your eyes and let your thoughts drift.

It's almost impossible to worry while lying in hot water, breathing in fragrant steam, with candle light and soft music playing. If this is too much for some guys, try a hot tub.

7. Remember Relaxation. It doesn't help if you step out of the bathroom after your spa and yell at the kids. All these techniques give you practice and an experience of what you're after all the time. It all

takes practice. You feel very calm after meditating; so hold on to that feeling as you go about your regular life. You feel as relaxed as a rag doll after you've layed on the floor and relaxed your entire body, so keep the feeling with you. Don't let things get to you. If you notice the stress building up, remember that relaxed feeling, and act from there.

8. Have fun. Have physical fun. Do things with your body. In my case, when I'm told I SHOULD do something (even when I'm the one doing the telling!) I get rebellious, and I resist doing it. So I tell myself I COULD. So give yourself permission to choose. When you allow your body to get physical it does feel so good!!!

9. Do what you love. Don't let your life go by without following your dreams. When you love what you do, it's a kind of relaxation. And you're not burdened by the stress of unfulfilled dreams. Even if you can't live your dreams all the time, at least make time for them. That can be enough. And then it's very possible that you will learn to love what you must do.

10. Make time for your friends and family. Never let your work come before those you love. Always be there for your loved ones. Consider the big picture to see where your deepest satisfaction lies, and live your life with no regrets.

You or someone you know can win the battle against ADD. The question is, how badly do you/they want to win?

A Helpful Tip: Schedule a time or two in your every day routine to relax. It can be as simple as breathing, taking a break from work or even meditating.

Thank you for reading my book, I truly hope my story and resources can assist you or someone you know.

Acknowledgements & ADD Resources

In my experience, I have found the following resources very beneficial in assisting me with overcoming the challenges of ADD. I would also like to acknowledge each of these resources and people have been a part of my life in the challenges I have faced with ADD. Thank you to all.

a) Kate Crosby
   Thank you for the honest read, editing and suggestions :)

b) Coaching
   Peter Quily, Vancouver BC,
   www.addcoach4u.com
   http://adultaddstrengths.com

c) Doctors
- Dr. Gabor Mate, Vancouver, BC
   http://drgabormate.com/
- Dr. Ed Hallowell, Boston, MA
   http://www.drhallowell.com/contact/index.cfm
- Dr. Frank Lawlis, Los Angeles, CA
   www.franklawlis.com
- Dr. Holly Prochnau, Ph.D., Coquitlam, BC
   604-464-1888

d) Web
   www.addcoach4u.com
   www.adultaddstrengths.com
   www.pillsdontteachskills.com
   www.scatteredminds.com/
   www.adhdnews.com
   www.add-adhd-help-center.com

http://www.drhallowell.com
http://www.add.about.com/
http://www.add.org/
www.help4adhd.org
www.adhdmarriage.com
www.totallyadd.com
www.caddac.ca
http://www.chadd.org/
http://www.chaddcanada.org/

e) Support Groups
- Vancouver Adult ADD Support Group Raven Song Community Health Centre at 2450 Ontario Street, Vancouver
- Directory of local ADD Support Groups can be Googled.
- List of ADHD Support Groups in Canada, the US, and Internationally can be found at http://www.addcoach4u.com/support/addsupportgroupresources.html

f) Recommended Books
- Delivered From Distraction by Dr. Ed Hallowell
- Scattered Minds by Dr. Gabor Mate The
- ADD Answer by DR. Frank Laless
- ADD-Friendly Ways to Organize Your Life by Judith Kolberg and Kathleen Nadeau
- Organizing Solutions for People with Attention Deficit Disorder by Susan C Pinsky

g) Recommended Video
Daniel Amen - Frazeled Parents